National Health Education Standards

THIRD EDITION

SHAPE AMERICA –
SOCIETY OF HEALTH AND PHYSICAL EDUCATORS

PRINCIPAL WRITERS

Kandice Porter, PhD, MCHES©

Holly Alperin, EdM, MCHES©

Angela Beale-Tawfeeq, PhD, MPH

Mary Connolly, MEd, CHES©

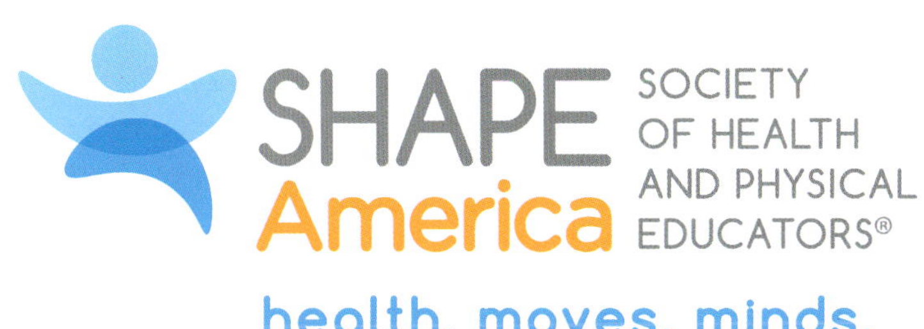

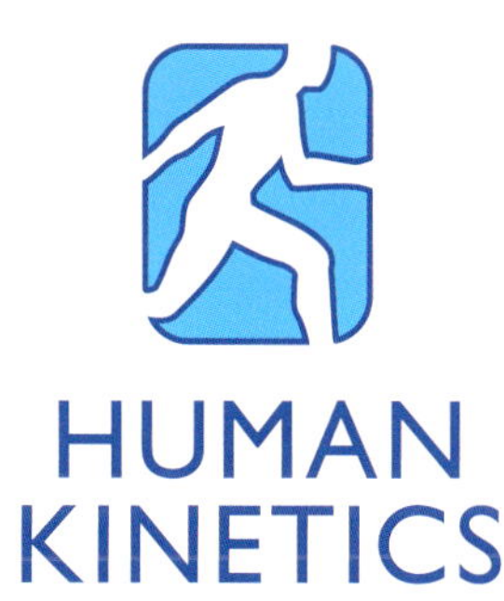

Library of Congress Cataloging-in-Publication Data

Names: SHAPE America (Organization), author.
Title: National health education standards / SHAPE America (Society of Health and Physical Educators) ; principal writers Kandice Porter, Holly Alperin, Angela Beale-Tawfeeq, Mary Connolly.
Description: Third edition. | Champaign, IL : Human Kinetics, 2025. | Revised edition of: National health education standards / developed by the Joint Committee on National Health Education Standards. Atlanta, Ga. : American Cancer Society, c2007. | Includes bibliographical references.
Identifiers: LCCN 2024004253 (print) | LCCN 2024004254 (ebook) | ISBN 9781718230682 (paperback) | ISBN 9781718230699 (epub) | ISBN 9781718230705 (pdf)
Subjects: LCSH: Health education--United States--Standards. | BISAC: EDUCATION / Teaching / Subjects / Health & Sexuality | EDUCATION / Teaching / Subjects / Physical Education
Classification: LCC RA440.3.U5 J65 2025 (print) | LCC RA440.3.U5 (ebook) | DDC 613.071--dc23/eng/20240129
LC record available at https://lccn.loc.gov/2024004253
LC ebook record available at https://lccn.loc.gov/2024004254

ISBN: 978-1-7182-3068-2 (print)

Permission notices for material reprinted in this book from other sources can be found on page 101.

The web addresses cited in this text were current as of February 2024, unless otherwise noted.

Acquisitions Editor: Bethany J. Bentley; **Managing Editor:** Anna Lan Seaman; **Copyeditor:** Marissa Wold Uhrina; **Proofreader:** Jen Swanson; **Permissions Managers:** Adam Pomerantz and Laurel Mitchell; **Senior Graphic Designers:** Nancy Rasmus and Joe Buck; **Cover Designer:** Keri Evans; **Cover Design Specialist:** Susan Rothermel Allen; **Photograph (cover):** FatCamera/E+/Getty Images; Courtney Hale/E+/Getty Images; Kali9/E+/Getty Images; **Photo Asset Manager:** Laura Fitch; **Photo Production Manager:** Jason Allen; **Senior Art Manager:** Kelly Hendren; **Illustrations:** © Human Kinetics, unless otherwise noted; **Printer:** Walsworth

Printed in the United States of America 10 9 8 7 6 5 4 3 2 1

The paper in this book was manufactured using responsible forestry methods.

Human Kinetics
1607 N. Market Street
Champaign, IL 61820
USA

United States and International
Website: **US.HumanKinetics.com**
Email: info@hkusa.com
Phone: 1-800-747-4457

Canada
Website: **Canada.HumanKinetics.com**
Email: info@hkcanada.com

SHAPE America – Society of Health and Physical Educators
PO Box 225
Annapolis Junction, MD 20701
Website: **www.shapeamerica.org**
Phone: 1-800-213-7193

E9563

CONTENTS

LETTER FROM THE CEO

SHAPE America is proud to champion and safeguard the 2024 SHAPE America National Health Education Standards, which serve as the foundation for a high-quality, school-based health education curriculum. As the Society of Health and Physical Educators—serving as the voice for more than 200,000 health and physical education professionals—SHAPE America is the nation's largest organization representing school-based health education professionals. We hold a deep commitment to this professional community and, as such, SHAPE America has proudly invested time and effort in producing many national resources and professional development opportunities for health education teachers.

SHAPE America was thrilled at the opportunity that arose in fall 2020 to maintain and champion copyright of the National Health Education Standards, including all derivatives and revisions, and to take on the long overdue work of updating the National HE Standards.

The National Health Education Standards Task Force, which is composed of innovative and diverse experts in school-based health education and represents leading national health education organizations, state departments of education, health education teacher preparation programs, and K-12 health educators, has worked tirelessly for over two years to bring the third edition of the National HE Standards to the field.

We are grateful and excited to be the organization most equipped to ensure the implementation and adoption of these standards by supporting school-based health educators through a robust suite of implementation resources and professional learning.

SHAPE America and our partners remain committed to the fact that the National HE Standards have, and always will be, the nation's health education standards.

Stephanie A. Morris
Chief Executive Officer, SHAPE America

PREFACE

Our Vision

Remembrance, reflection, reimagining, and unforgetting are concepts that, like a spool of thread, have been used to weave together the narratives of communities with the goal of deepening the understanding of the connection between one's history and its connection to present-day issues affecting a community (Beale-Tawfeeq et. al, 2023; Kendi & Macy, 2023; Krawec, 2022; Bhattacharya et al., 2020; Antonovsky, 1996). We use these concepts as a guiding force in our efforts to explore why health education is essential and to remember our children, families, and communities.

We live in a time when school-based health education has dedicated itself to achieving a vision: of becoming a nation where children and adolescents are healthy, fit, and ready to learn; where youth are prepared with essential skills needed to live life to its fullest; where adult health and **wellness** are the natural outgrowth of skills, understanding, and behavior built from childhood; and where health challenges and differences in race, culture, background, ability, and socioeconomic status do not prevent our most precious human resources from reaching their potential (CDC, 2019, 2023; Kendi & Macy, 2023; Krawec, 2023; Learning for Justice, n.d.; Bhattacharya et al., 2020; Benes & Alperin, 2022; Benes, 2020; Persaud et al., 2021; Delpit, 2012; American Cancer Society, 2007; Antonovsky, 1996). We must imagine a nation where children and adolescents are wise about the influences of technology and the media on their lives; where they are prepared to be prudent consumers of goods and services that enhance their health and well-being; where they are skilled in employing thoughtful decision-making and goal-setting strategies to achieve their greatest ambitions; and where they passionately and compassionately advocate for the best for themselves, their families, and their communities (Office of Disease Prevention and Health Promotion, n.d.; American Cancer Society, 2007; Antonovsky, 1996; Bhattacharya et al., 2020; Benes, 2019; Benes & Alperin, 2022; Kendi & Macy, 2023; Krawec, 2023; Learning for Justice, 2023; Persaud et al., 2021).

As health educators, we must believe in this vision, remember that effective advocacy requires the understanding of these complex contexts, and strive to create school-based health education programs that support the development of health literacy, competence, and self-efficacy skills. Through the use of the National HE Standards, we can make this an attainable goal for our children and for all of the generations to come.

"'A'ohe hana nui ke alu 'ia."

"No task is too big when done together by all."

Hawaiian proverb

STATEMENT OF SUPPORT FROM THE AMERICAN FEDERATION OF TEACHERS

Students enter school with a vast array of social, emotional, physical, and academic needs. SHAPE America's effort to update the National Health Education Standards and the National Physical Education Standards is a crucial part of the work to address these needs and improve children's well-being. The new standards bolster students' learning by doing; skills-based health education best equips students to lead active and healthy lifelong wellness journeys.

Educators across the nation face deprofessionalization and demoralization—we see it and fight it daily. The AFT applauds SHAPE America for understanding that educators today need a culture of collaboration, proper teaching and learning conditions, and real voice and agency. Inclusive task forces worked deliberately and thoughtfully to develop the updated National HE Standards and National PE Standards through admirably open and iterative engagement. As a result, the new standards reflect educators' commitment to real solutions for children's well-being.

Randi Weingarten
President, American Federation of Teachers

ACKNOWLEDGMENTS

The revision of the 2024 SHAPE America National Health Education Standards would not have been possible without the time, dedication, and effort of the revision task force, reviewers in the field, and educators who will eventually use these standards. SHAPE America wishes to sincerely thank and acknowledge the National HE Standards Revision Task Force members.

Nadine Marchessault, MEd, NBCT, Co-chair
Hawai'i Department of Education

Sarah Toth, PhD, MEd, MCHES©, Co-chair
Alabama Agricultural and Mechanical University

Holly Alperin, EdM, MCHES©
University of New Hampshire

Angela Beale-Tawfeeq, PhD, MPH
Rowan University

Laurie Bechhofer, MPH
Michigan Department of Education

Mary Connolly, MEd, CHES©
Cambridge College

Nana Donkor, MS
Prince George's County Public Schools, Maryland

Angela Glymph, PhD
Peer Health Exchange

Jamie Hurley, PhD, MEd
Colorado Department of Education

Michelle Westerling Ireland, MA, MCHES©
Hanover Public Schools, Massachusetts

Kaulana Molina, MS, NBCT
Punahou School, Hawai'i

Kandice Porter, PhD, MCHES©
Kennesaw State University

Tilsa Rodriguez-Gonzalez
City School District of New Rochelle, New York

Andrew Snyder, MAT
Nevada Department of Education

Erin Sweeney, PhD, MEd, MCHES©
University of Nebraska at Kearney

Leigh Szucs, PhD, CHES©
Centers for Disease Control and Prevention

In addition to the task force members, hundreds of individuals and many groups provided feedback through invited reviews, town halls, coffee talks, presentations, and surveys throughout this process.

Thank you to the SHAPE America Health Education Council; the National Physical Education Standards Task Force; the Equity, Diversity, and Inclusion Committee; and the Health and Physical Education State and District Administrators Special Interest Group for your engagement in the revision process.

Finally, thank you to all who participated in this process by contributing your thoughtful expertise and experience to develop standards to serve as the foundational framework for school-based health education throughout the country.

CHAPTER 1

Introduction

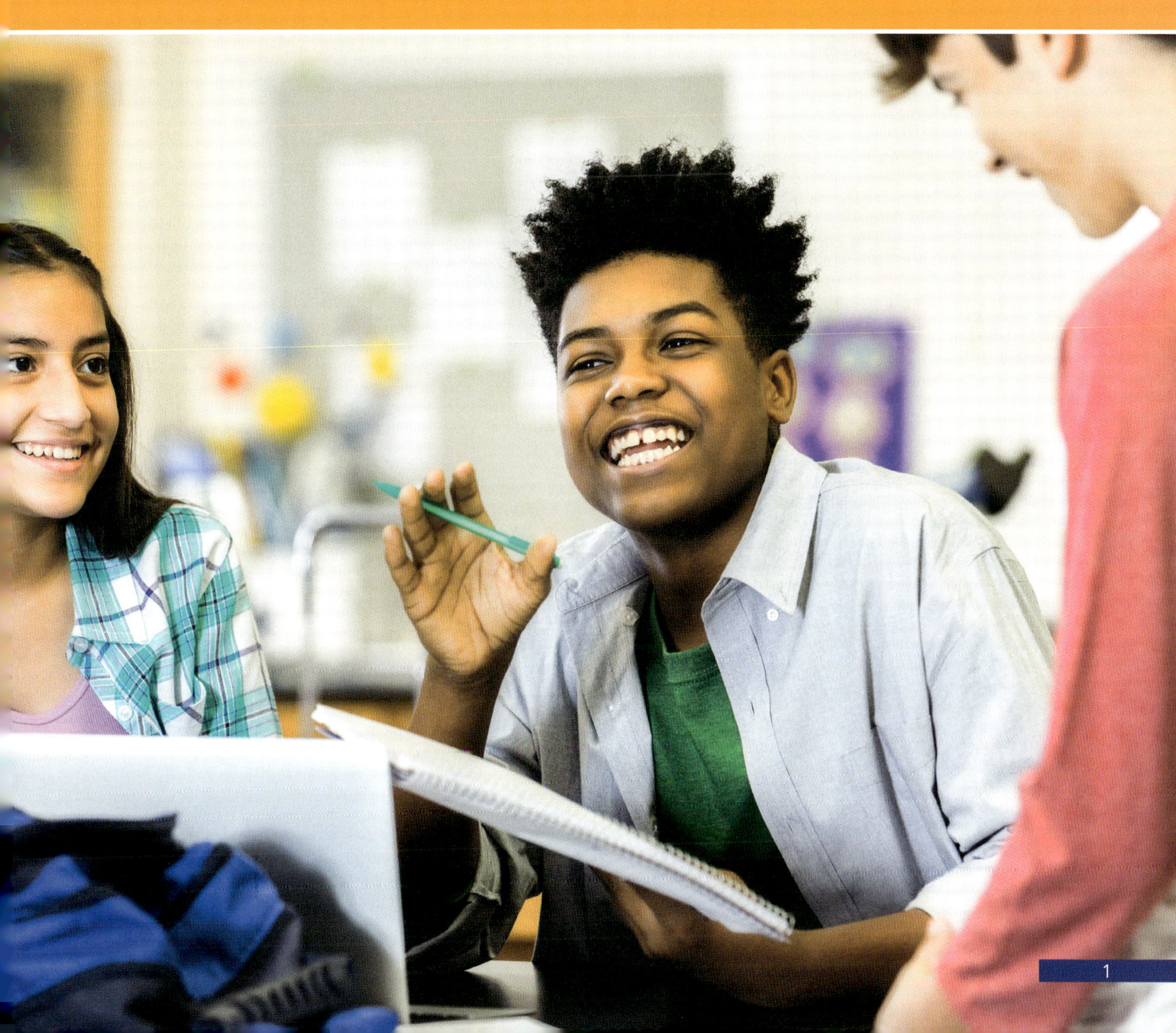

Starting With "Why" and Realizing "How"

"Health is a state of optimal physical, mental and social well-being and not merely the absence of disease and infirmity."

World Health Organization (WHO; n.d.)

The goal of health education is to provide students with the knowledge and skills needed to lead healthy lifestyles, and a skills-based approach is a best practice for delivering high-quality health education. It is the intent of the 2024 SHAPE America National Health Education Standards to serve as a framework designed to provide multiple layers of support to health education stakeholders (i.e., preK-12 health educators and administrators; families and caregivers; health education teacher education [HETE]; higher education professional preparation programs [HEPPP]; community-based organizations, agencies, institutions, and businesses [CBOAIB]; non-governmental agencies [NGO]; local and state education agencies [LEA] [SEA]; national organizations and agencies [NOA]; and policymakers). Health education, when implemented through the framework of the National Health Education Standards, provides students with the essential tools, knowledge, and skills needed to support their personal health and to address the historical and current structural issues that affect health (CDC, 2019, 2023; Kendi & Macy, 2023; Persaud et al, 2021; Benes, 2019). Therefore, to frame the work of health educators and health education stakeholders, let us remember to start with "why" and to use this revised edition of the National HE Standards to provide students, families, and communities with concrete expectations for health education.

The efforts taken to revise and reimagine the current National HE Standards framework were not taken lightly nor approached with ease, and it is with this goal of health education in mind that the revised standards reflect the diverse and collective voices that contributed to this intentional process (see chapter 7, Background on Standards Development). The voices of many health educators were heard as a charge for us all to engage in this coordinated effort, to remember our "why," and to strive through our professional actions to use the revised National HE Standards as a foundation for the following:

- Aligning, designing, or selecting curricula and allocating instructional resources
- Providing a basis of assessment of students' achievement and progress (American Cancer Society, 2007)
- Providing equitable access to high-level, meaningful, and engaging health education for every student, family, and community regardless of race, color, national origin, ancestry, sex, gender identity, gender expression, sexual orientation, age, disability, and religion (U.S. Department of Justice, 2023; U.S. Equal Employment Opportunity Commission, 2023)

As a result, the revised standards reflect the following key shifts:

- They incorporate developmentally appropriate progressions of performance indicators for each standard across the grade spans.
- They incorporate **asset-based**, or **strength-based**, language (i.e., words, phrases, and concepts that focus on the strengths and potentials of students).
- They emphasize not only individual behavior change but also broader structures, including families, communities, and laws and policies that affect **health** and **well-being**.
- They incorporate themes related to advancing **diversity**, **equity**, **inclusion**, and social justice.

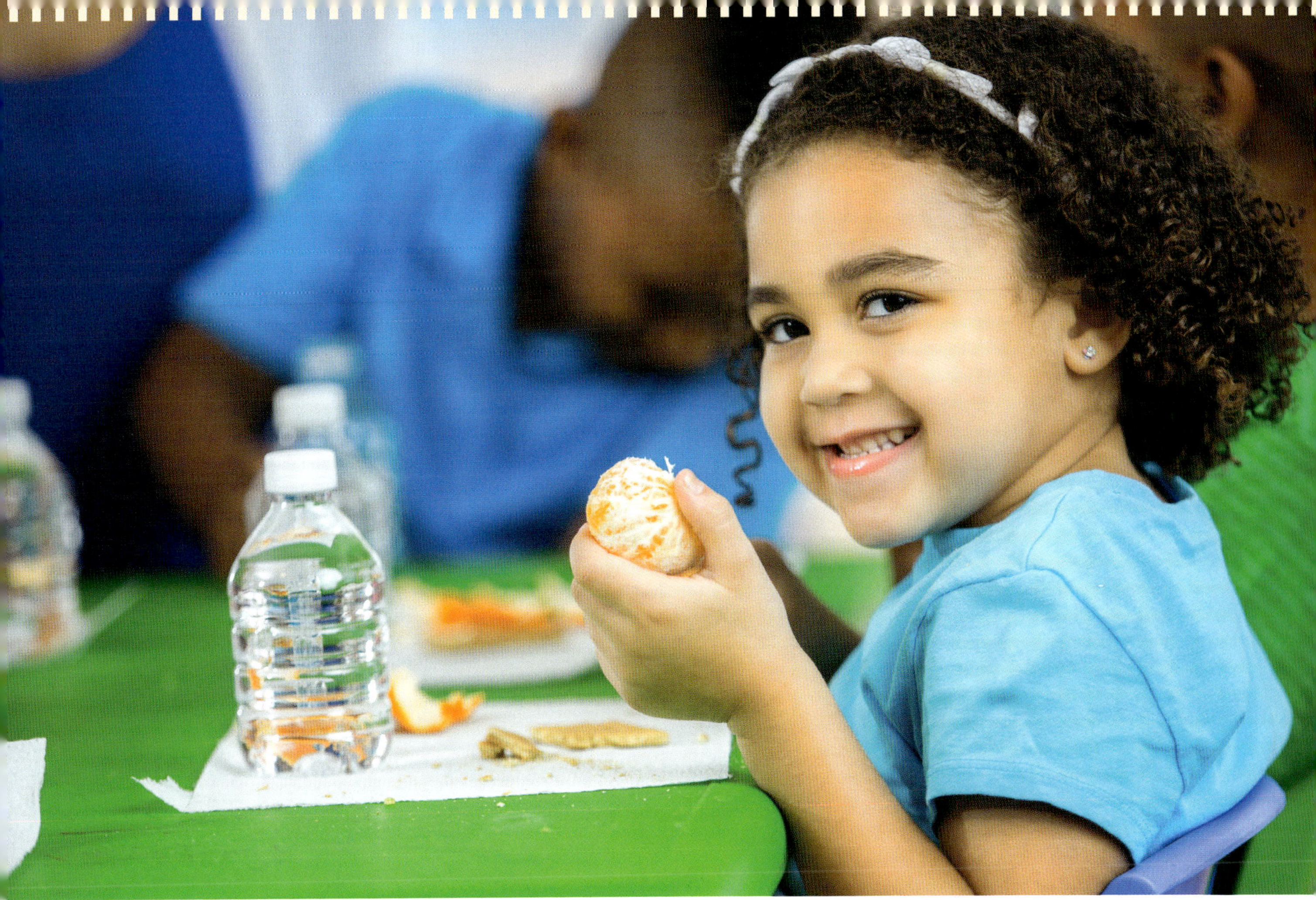

Our Call to Action: A Global Vision

Our role as health educators is to teach students that no knowledge is more crucial than knowledge about health and well-being. Without it, no other life goal can be achieved (Joint Committee, 2007; Boyer, 1990). We must remember the multiple critical events that have affected our country and have placed us all at an intersection of social change.

In January 2020 we all became a part of a global pandemic that lives in our collective memory. For SHAPE America, this time also renewed a call to action, one that provided the opportunity for SHAPE America to revise the National HE Standards. The revised edition of the National HE Standards has an increased focus on behavior theory and supports health educators in exploring a strengths-based approach to health education, which helps students "build from and strengthen their assets" (Benes & Alperin, 2022; SHAPE America, 2022). The revision of the National HE Standards encourages health educators and health education stakeholders to embrace the critical role that school-based preK-12 health education provides in supporting the "conditions in which people are born, live, learn, work, play, worship, and age," known as the **social determinants of health (SDOH)** (see figure 1.1; U.S. Department of Health and Human Services, Office of Disease Prevention and Health Promotion, 2018) and in supporting the national goals of improving health and well-being as outlined in Healthy People 2030. (Health education–related objectives from Healthy People 2030 can be found in appendix B.)

Social Determinants of Health
Education Access and Quality
Health Care Access and Quality
Economic Stability
Neighborhood and Built Environment
Social and Community Context

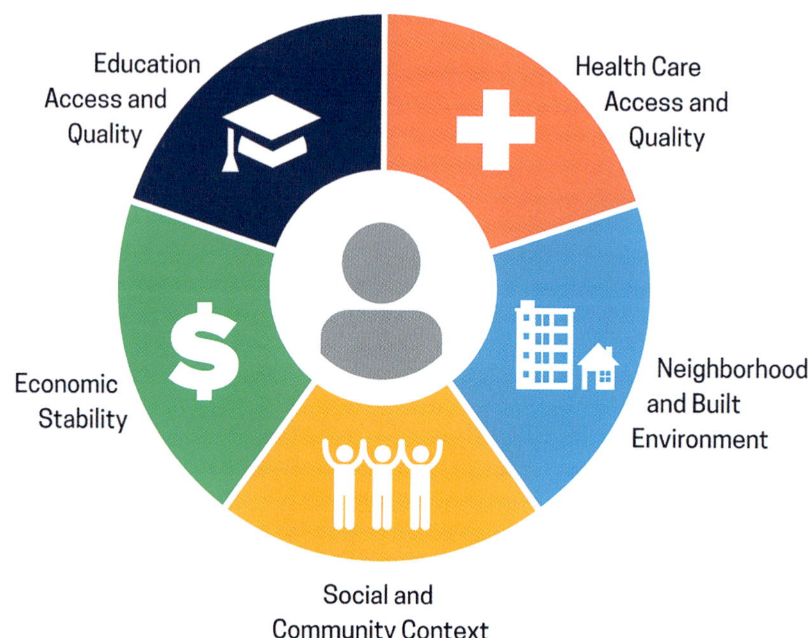

FIGURE 1.1 Social determinants of health (SDOH).
From CDC (2023).

"America faces three major crises right now, a viral pandemic the likes of which we have not seen since 1918, an economic collapse the likes of which we have not seen since 1932 at the onset of the Great Depression, and the ongoing expressions of the struggle of civil rights and equity, the likes of which we have not seen since 1968. These are synergistic conditions, which in tandem have enormous implications for public health. They expose the continuing problem of injustice, inequality, and structural and systemic racism in America."

ASPPH (2020, p. 1)

In the United States these synergistic conditions have had enormous implications for public health. Health education is more crucial now than ever. School-aged youth, families, and communities are experiencing unprecedented geopolitical and global unrest, national and environmental fragility, discrimination, racism, income and wealth inequality, and systems of education that challenge the rights of all school-aged youth to be provided with equitable opportunities for high-level, meaningful, and engaging learning experiences (ASPPH, 2020; CDC, 2020; Persaud et al., 2021; Benes, 2019; Benes & Alperin, 2022). Schools need the infrastructure, provided by this revised edition of the National HE Standards, to support health educators, administrators, and health education stakeholders in their ability to design or select the best health education curricula and to provide all school-aged youth with high-quality health education that will empower them to be health-literate change agents in their own lives, communities, and the broader social context of the world.

What Is Worth Doing

What is worth doing in school health education, in our classrooms and communities, to engage our students, support our families, connect with our communities, and change and save lives?

It is the intent that the revised National HE Standards be used to support the effective implementation of integrated models that promote health and well-being, such as the **Whole School, Whole Community, Whole Child (WSCC) model** (see figure 1.2). The WSCC model places the child at the center and takes a collaborative, comprehensive, multisectoral approach to support learning. With the use of

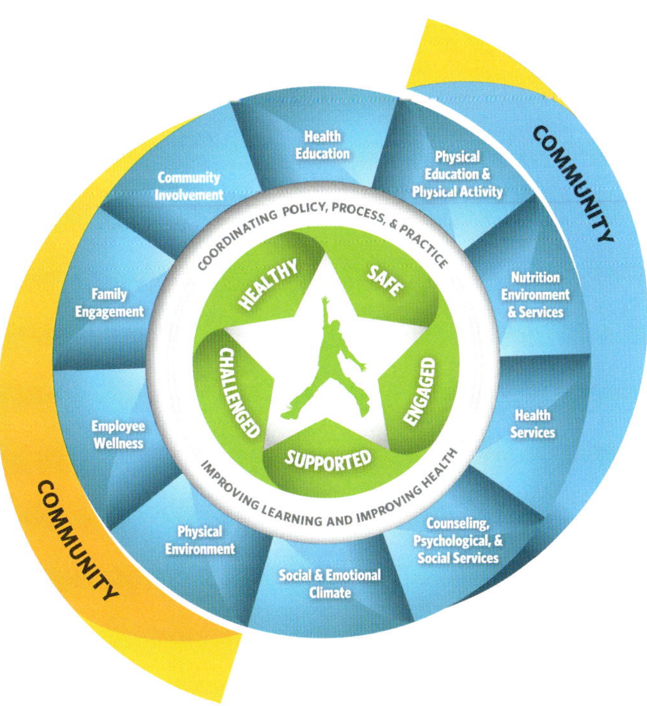

FIGURE 1.2 The Whole School, Whole Community, Whole Child model promotes health and well-being.

Adapted by permission from Whole School, Whole Community, Whole Child model, (Arlington, VA: ASCD. © 2005), 7. All rights reserved.

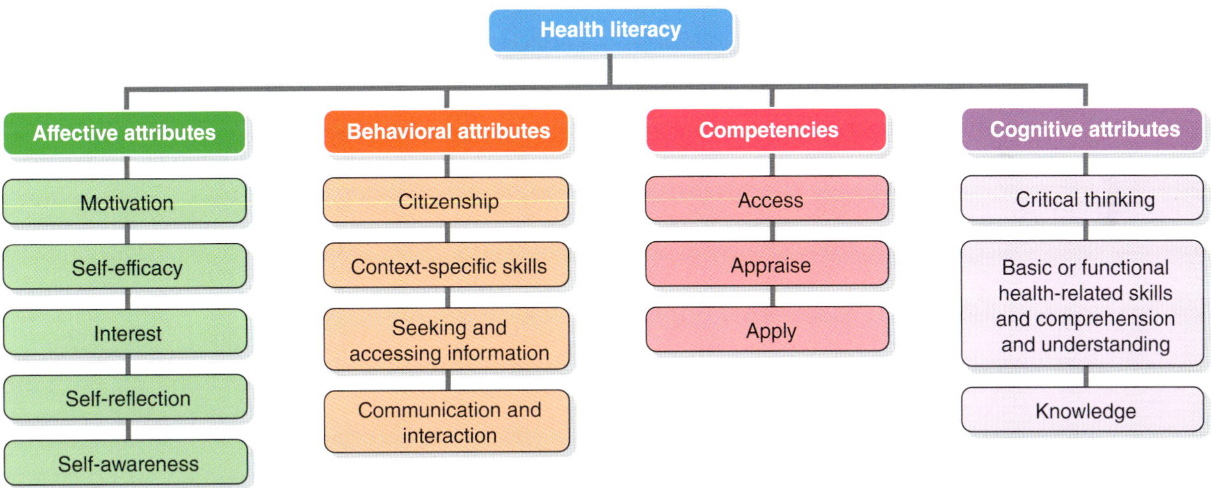

FIGURE 1.3 Components of health literacy are necessary assets that influence a student's health and well-being.

Reprinted by permission from S. Benes and H. Alperin, *The Essentials of Teaching Health Education: Curriculum, Instruction and Assessment*, 2nd ed. (Champaign, IL: Human Kinetics, 2022).

the revised National HE Standards, and grounded in WSCC, schools have a vital role in supporting the development of **health literacy** as an asset and valuable quality that can help students feel empowered with the knowledge and skills to make health-enhancing choices, improve their health outcomes, and apply their health literacy to have agency in their lives (see figure 1.3; Benes & Alperin, 2022; USDHHS, 2018; Benes, 2019; Lewallen et al., 2015).

CHAPTER 2

Guiding Principles

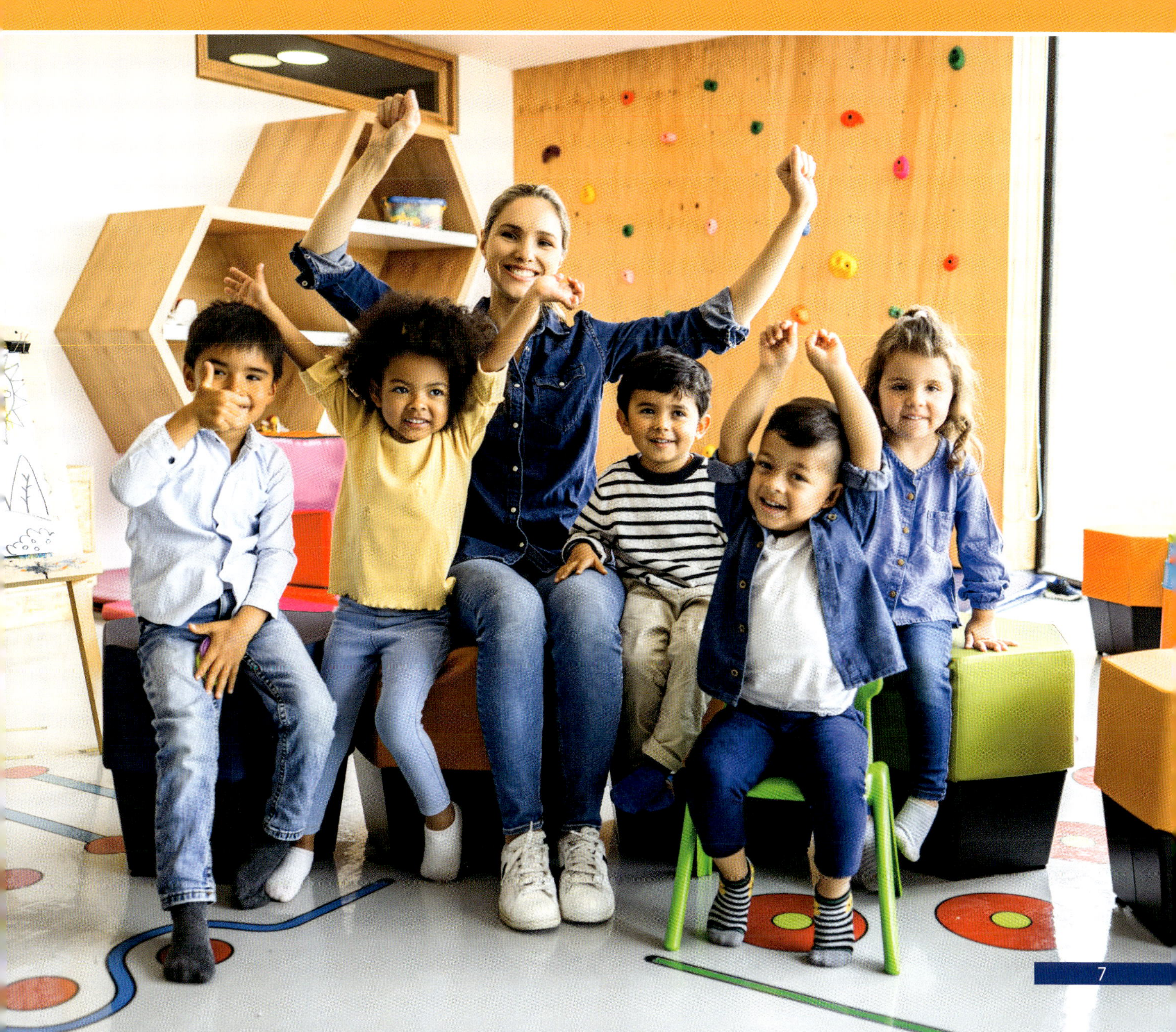

Health education is an opportunity to teach young people the knowledge and skills that can improve the health and well-being of themselves and others. It can also be an opportunity to support the journey of self-discovery, development of self-identity, and building positive relationships (Benes & Alperin, 2022, 2023).

It has long been an aim of the 2024 SHAPE America National Health Education Standards to support "all students to learn to make safe, appropriate, and healthful choices" (Joint Committee, 2007, p. 53). As such, it is necessary to provide students with classroom time to practice applying the skills and information they have learned in ways that maintain or improve their health and well-being within the context of authentic and real-world settings (SHAPE America, 2018).

"The goal of health education should contribute directly to a student's ability to successfully practice behaviors that protect and promote health."

American Cancer Society (2007)

When students deepen their knowledge of and skills in health education, they may experience potential benefits to their overall health and well-being. For example, developing the ability to determine what health information is valid and reliable is a critical component of being able to select health products and services that are most appropriate for individual needs, and being able to advocate for reducing stigma associated with mental illness or challenging mental health situations can be a key factor in creating a culture that provides support for mental health. However, the benefits also extend to the positive relationship between health outcomes and academic success (Cabrera et al., 2018; Centers for Disease Control and Prevention, 2014; Ickovics et al., 2014; Michael et al, 2015; Rasberry et al, 2015). Health education should be taught as an academic subject that is a required part of the overall curriculum and is considered a critical component of a well-rounded education (Office of Elementary and Secondary Education, 2016).

Finally, the skills and information taught in health education have a direct connection to many areas of the school and curriculum. In addition to health education courses, teachers should encourage direct connections to opportunities within the school building that support and bolster the health and well-being of young people. Various models exist that promote health and well-being across the school and connect with families and communities. For example, both the Whole School, Whole Community, Whole Child model (Centers for Disease Control and Prevention, 2023) and Health Promoting Schools (World Health Organization, 2019) encourage school personnel to integrate health and well-being across the whole building and to create a culture that supports the health and well-being of young people and adults in the building and surrounding community, fostering a sense of belonging and meaningful connections to people and places. Specific connections can include working with school health services, school nutrition services, or mental and emotional health services to ensure that similar health messaging is used throughout the school and that families are engaged in ways that transfer learning from the classroom to make connections at home. Seek out opportunities to connect to the physical education curriculum or to use community programming and resources that are available to support the needs of young people. Additionally, the standards taught in health education can be highlighted and promoted through various school-level initiatives and programming (examples of Action Steps for Implementation can be found in appendix A).

National Health Education Standards and Performance Indicators

This third edition of the National HE Standards is guided by prominent health behavior theories, including the socioecological model and the social cognitive theory, with the following underlying parameters used to form a foundation for the development of the standards and **performance indicators**:

- Health is a result of complex interactions at a variety of levels (personal, interpersonal, community, and society). As such, students must learn about health and ways to improve health across a variety of settings and situations.
- Research-based practice and understandings have been used to guide the development of the standards and performance indicators.
- Achieving health and well-being is the product of both individual and collective actions. While individuals have choice and free will, collectively individuals create social norms, laws, policies, and other systems that can help or hinder health and well-being. Therefore, any consideration of health and well-being must include analysis of the role that individuals play in the health outcomes of the collective community and recognize that individual actions have the potential to help or harm other members of a community.
- An emphasis on health and well-being forms the foundation for the National HE Standards. This allows learners to examine how to maintain or improve health and well-being along with reducing risk factors that may lead to adverse health outcomes for self or others.
- Skill development and application are the cornerstones for engaging in health behaviors that can positively affect health and well-being. The National HE Standards are designed to support skill development and meaningful application in a variety of settings.
- Health topics and content are always changing; as such, the specific integration of health content is determined at the local level.
- Health occurs across a variety of dimensions (e.g., physical, social, emotional, financial, intellectual, multicultural, environmental, spiritual), and it is vital that young people examine various dimensions of health and well-being as they pertain to their own lives and lived experiences (see figure 2.1).
- Focus on how building functional health knowledge and essential personal and social skills contributes directly to health outcomes.
- Developmental progression is built into the performance indicators, and while they are noted within grade spans, students may be at a different developmental level. Thus, it is important to use performance standards that are appropriate for the audiences and their contexts.

Spiritual
(relating to the meaning and purpose of life)
Emotional and mental
(relating to understanding oneself)
Social
(relating to relationships)
Environmental
(relating to the Earth and physical space)
Sexual
(relating to intimate partner relationships)
Health and wellness
Financial
(relating to money and socioeconomics)
Physical
(relating to the body)
Intellectual
(relating to lifelong learning)
Occupational
(relating to vocation or job)
Multicultural
(relating to learning about others)

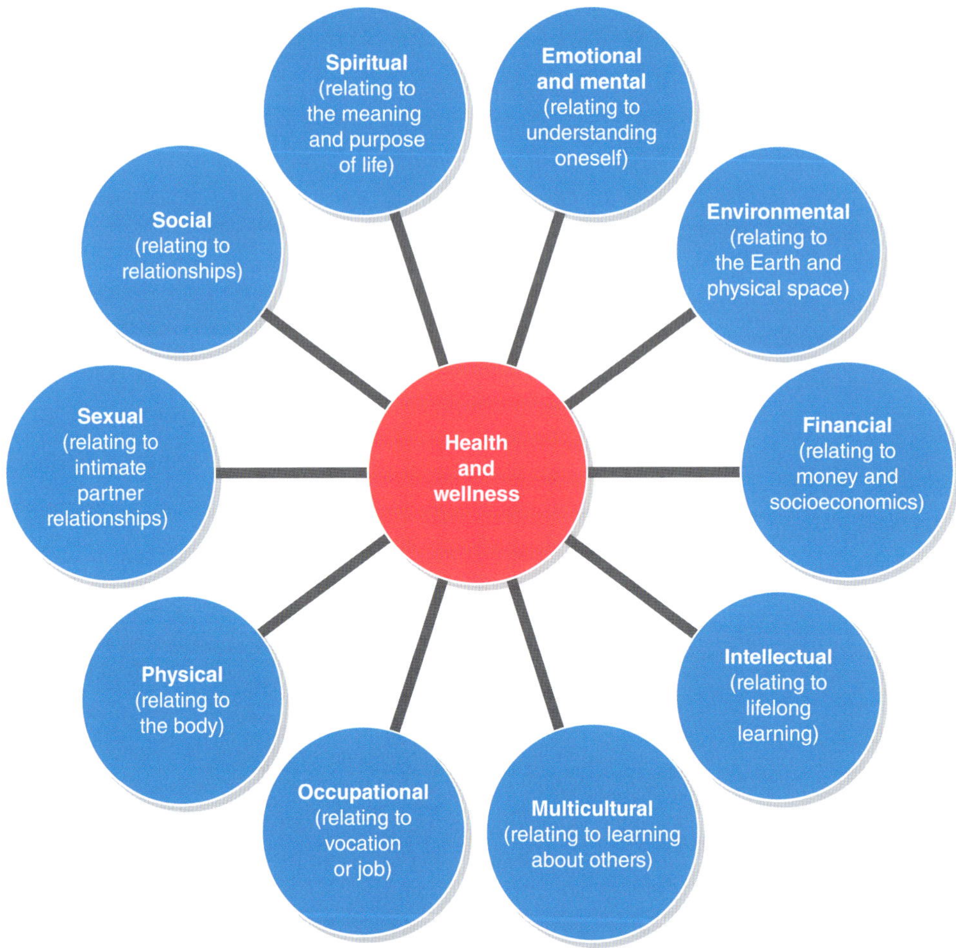

FIGURE 2.1 Dimensions of health.

Reprinted by permission from S. Benes and H. Alperin, *The Essentials of Teaching Health Education: Curriculum, Instruction and Assessment*, 2nd ed. (Champaign, IL: Human Kinetics, 2022).

Supporting Effective Implementation

To establish consistency throughout the document, the National Health Education Standards Revision Task Force operated under the following set of assumptions that are drawn from current research and theory in the field. These guiding principles emphasize two categories: the role and purpose of health education and curriculum, instruction, and assessment.

Role and Purpose of Health Education

1. Health education that is strengths based and asset focused is more effective in supporting behavior change and positive health outcomes.
2. Academic achievement and health status are interrelated.
3. Health education is one component of school-wide and community-wide efforts to address student health and well-being.

4. Each student, regardless of identity, ability, or development, deserves the opportunity to achieve personal health and well-being. Learning experiences in health education must honor and affirm the assets students bring to the table.
5. Environment has a substantial impact on an individual's health and well-being. Standards must encourage students to examine the variety of ways that the environment is a factor in health and health outcomes. Each student has a role to play in their surrounding environment and has an opportunity to positively affect the health and well-being of their communities.
6. Improvements in health outcomes can positively affect health care costs (Teisberg et al., 2020).
7. Effective health education can contribute to the establishment of a healthy and productive citizenry.

Curriculum, Instruction, and Assessment

1. Local curriculum planners should develop a curriculum that is based on local student needs.
2. Health education emphasizes skill development while integrating functional health information that supports young people's ability to adopt, practice, and maintain health and well-being.
3. Instruction by qualified and licensed health education teachers is essential for student achievement of the National HE Standards in school-based settings.
4. Sufficient instructional time is necessary to influence health behavior and health outcomes.
5. Students need opportunities to engage in cooperative and active learning strategies, including practice and reinforcement.
6. Students need multiple opportunities and a variety of assessment strategies to determine achievement of health standards and performance indicators.

Characteristics of Effective Health Education Curricula

Characteristics of Effective Health Education Curricula (CDC, 2019) provides additional guidance in the creation of the third edition of the National HE Standards and in supporting integration of these standards at the local, programmatic level. These characteristics are grounded in professional literature that has been examined and synthesized with input from experts in the field of health education. Many of the following characteristics are reflected in both the standards and the performance indicators.

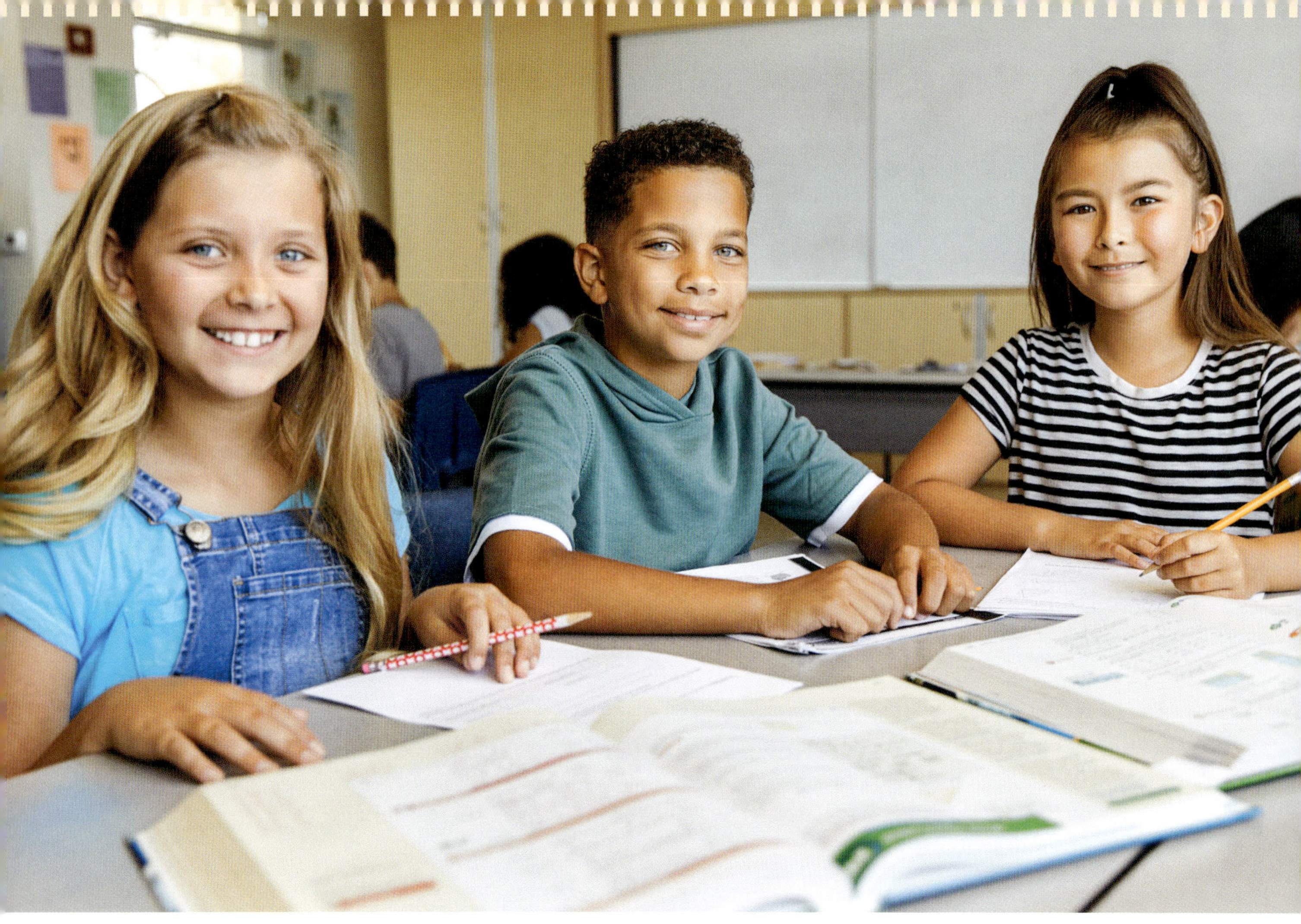

An effective health education curriculum achieves the following:

- It focuses on clear health goals and related behavioral outcomes.

  An effective curriculum has clear health-related goals and behavioral outcomes that are directly related to these goals. Instructional strategies and learning experiences are directly related to the behavioral outcomes.

- It is research based and theory driven.

  An effective curriculum has instructional strategies and learning experiences built on theoretical approaches (e.g., social cognitive theory and social inoculation theory) that have effectively influenced health-related behaviors among youth. The most promising curriculum goes beyond the cognitive level and addresses health determinants, social factors, attitudes, values, norms, and skills that influence specific health-related behaviors.

- It addresses individual values, attitudes, and beliefs.

  An effective curriculum fosters attitudes, **values**, and beliefs that support positive health behaviors. It provides instructional strategies and learning experiences that motivate students to critically examine personal perspectives, thoughtfully consider new arguments that support health-promoting attitudes and values, and generate positive perceptions about protective behaviors and negative perceptions about risk behaviors.

- It focuses on reinforcing **protective factors** and increasing perceptions of personal risk and harmfulness of engaging in specific unhealthy practices and behaviors.

  An effective curriculum provides opportunities for students to validate positive health-promoting beliefs, intentions, and behaviors. It provides opportunities for students to assess their vulnerability to health problems, actual risk of engaging in harmful health behaviors, and exposure to unhealthy situations.

- It addresses social pressures and influences.

  An effective curriculum provides opportunities for students to analyze personal and social pressures to engage in risky behaviors, such as media influence, peer pressure, and social barriers.

- It builds personal competence, social competence, and self-efficacy by addressing skills.

  An effective curriculum builds essential skills—including communication, refusal, assessing accuracy of information, decision-making, planning and goal-setting, self-control, and self-management—that enable students to build their personal confidence, deal with social pressures, and avoid or reduce risk behaviors.

  For each skill, students are guided through a series of developmental steps:

  - Discussing the importance of the skill, its relevance, and its relationship to other learned skills
  - Presenting steps for developing the skill
  - Modeling the skill
  - Practicing and rehearsing the skill using real-life scenarios
  - Providing feedback and reinforcement

- It provides functional health knowledge that is basic and accurate and directly contributes to health-promoting decisions and behaviors.

  An effective curriculum provides accurate, reliable, and credible information for usable purposes so that students can assess risk, clarify attitudes and beliefs, correct misperceptions about social norms, identify ways to avoid or minimize risky situations, examine internal and external influences, make behaviorally relevant decisions, and build personal and social competence. A curriculum that provides information for the sole purpose of improving knowledge of factual information will not change behavior.

- It uses strategies designed to personalize information and engage students.

  An effective curriculum includes instructional strategies and learning experiences that are student centered, interactive, and experiential (e.g., group discussions, cooperative learning, problem-solving, role-playing, and peer-led activities). Learning experiences correspond with students' cognitive and emotional development, help them personalize information, and maintain their interest and motivation while accommodating diverse capabilities and learning styles. Instructional strategies and learning experiences include methods for the following:

- › Addressing key health-related concepts
- › Encouraging creative expression
- › Sharing personal thoughts, feelings, and opinions
- › Thoughtfully considering new arguments
- › Developing critical thinking skills

- It provides age-appropriate and **developmentally appropriate** information, learning strategies, teaching methods, and materials.

  An effective curriculum addresses students' needs, interests, concerns, developmental and emotional maturity levels, experiences, and current knowledge and skill levels. Learning is relevant and applicable to students' daily lives. Concepts and skills are covered in a logical sequence.

- It incorporates learning strategies, teaching methods, and materials that are culturally inclusive.

  An effective curriculum has materials that are free of culturally biased information but includes information, activities, and examples that are inclusive of diverse cultures and lifestyles (e.g., gender, race, ethnicity, religion, age, physical and mental ability, appearance, and sexual orientation). Strategies promote values, attitudes, and behaviors that acknowledge the cultural diversity of students, optimize relevance to students from multiple cultures in the school community, strengthen students' skills needed to engage in intercultural interactions, and build on the cultural resources of families and communities.

- It provides adequate time for instruction and learning.

  An effective curriculum provides enough time to promote understanding of key health concepts and practice skills. Behavior change requires an intensive and sustained effort. A short-term or one-shot curriculum, delivered for a few hours at one grade level, is generally insufficient to support the adoption and maintenance of healthy behaviors.

- It provides opportunities to reinforce skills and positive health behaviors.

  An effective curriculum builds on previously learned concepts and skills and provides opportunities to reinforce health-promoting skills across health topics and grade levels. This can include incorporating more than one practice application of a skill, adding skill-booster sessions at subsequent grade levels, or integrating skill application opportunities in other academic areas. A curriculum that addresses age-appropriate determinants of behavior across grade levels and reinforces and builds on learning is more likely to achieve longer-lasting results.

- It provides opportunities to make positive connections with influential others.

  An effective curriculum links students to influential persons who affirm and reinforce health-promoting norms, attitudes, values, beliefs, and behaviors. Instructional strategies build on protective factors that promote healthy behaviors and enable students to avoid or reduce health risk behaviors by engaging peers, parents, families, and other positive adult role models in student learning.

- It includes teacher information and plans for professional development and training that enhance effectiveness of instruction and student learning.

An effective curriculum is implemented by teachers who have a personal interest in promoting positive health behaviors, believe in what they are teaching, are knowledgeable about the curriculum content, and are comfortable and skilled in implementing expected instructional strategies. Ongoing professional development and training is critical for helping teachers implement a new curriculum or strategies that require new skills in teaching or assessment.

Health Education Through a Skills-Based Approach

The National HE Standards are designed with one standard (Standard 1) that emphasizes the application and acquisition of functional health information. The remaining seven standards (Standards 2-8) focus on students increasing their ability to use and apply health skills in authentic and meaningful ways. The emphasis on skill development within the National HE Standards supports students in developing the ability to work actively toward health and well-being at any age. This emphasis on skill development in health education is referred to as a *skills-based approach.*

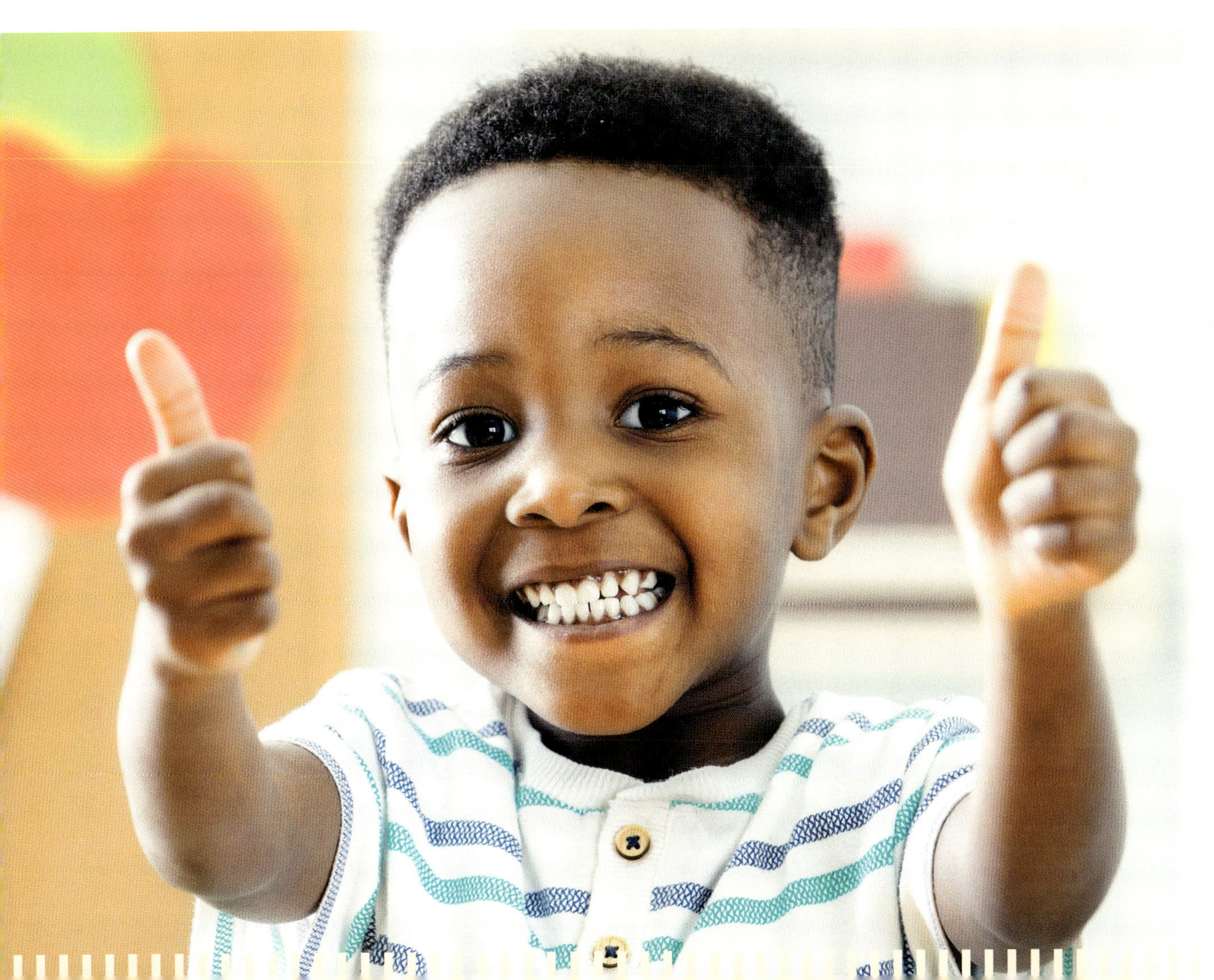

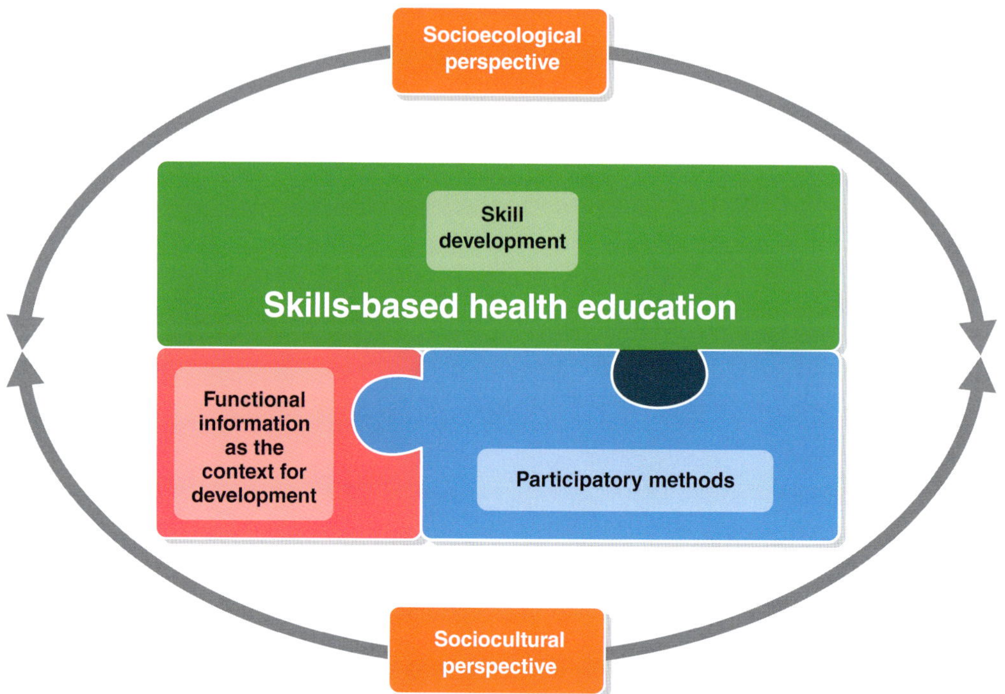

FIGURE 2.2 Key aspects of skills-based approach.

Reprinted by permission from S. Benes and H. Alperin, *The Essentials of Teaching Health Education: Curriculum, Instruction and Assessment*, 2nd ed. (Champaign, IL: Human Kinetics, 2022).

A skills-based approach can be defined as a

> planned, sequential, comprehensive, and relevant set of learning experiences implemented through socioecological and sociocultural perspectives and participatory methods in order to support the development of skills, attitudes, and functional knowledge needed to maintain, enhance, or promote the health and well-being of self and others across multiple **dimensions of wellness**. (Benes & Alperin, 2022)

By following this definition of a skills-based approach, educators are encouraged to teach health education in a way that honors and affirms each learner and allows time for students to use and practice the skills that will support their own health and well-being along with the health and well-being of others around them and in the community (see figure 2.2). Additionally, a skills-based approach is supported by brain research. When we create a space for students to learn in a collaborative, safe learning environment, we support the adolescent brain's desire to "seek and find" (Connolly, 2020; Wolfe, 2001). When learners have a deliberate opportunity to develop new skills that support their health and well-being, they become active participants in the development of health literacy across many levels.

Collectively, a variety of theories, guiding principles, and practices influenced the design of this edition. As such, it is encouraged that educators implementing these standards consider the broader and deeper implications to the health and well-being of individuals and communities. Those implementing the National HE Standards are encouraged to share the standards with colleagues, stakeholders, and partners who are engaged in complementary work.

CHAPTER 3

Equity, Access, and Inclusion for Each Student

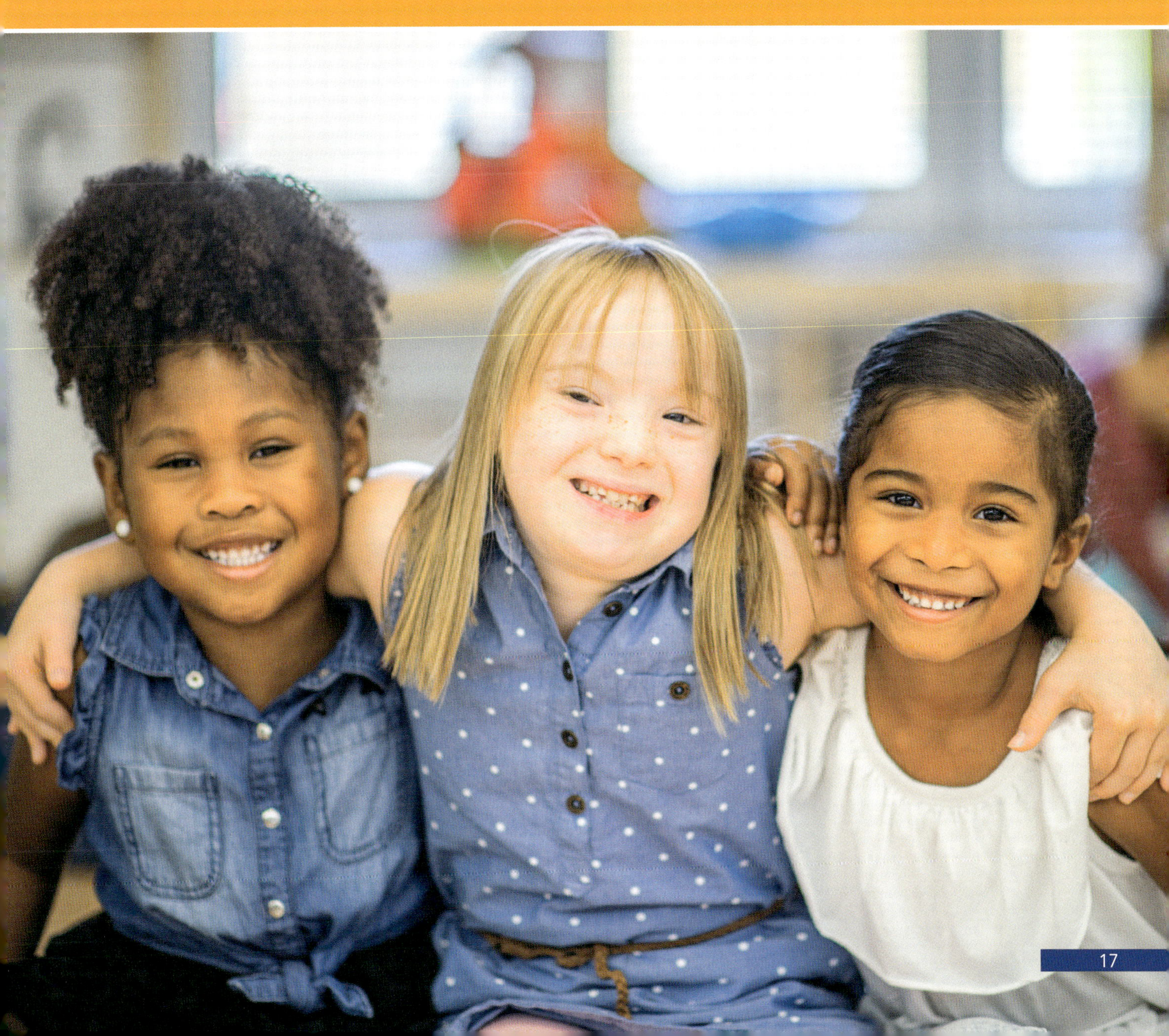

"Let's invite one another in. Maybe then we can begin to fear less, to make fewer wrong assumptions, to let go of the biases and stereotypes that unnecessarily divide us. Maybe we can better embrace the ways we are the same."

Michelle Obama

Globally, and in the United States, incidents of discrimination, social exclusion, and prejudice have left few health educators feeling prepared to incorporate a curriculum that is **culturally responsive** and humanizing for students, thus compromising students' well-being and resulting in low academic achievement, negative health outcomes, and injury (Kendi & Macy, 2023; Benes & Alperin, 2022; Tai et al., 2022; Persaud et al., 2021; Culp, 2021; Benes, 2019; Killen & Rutland, 2022; Delpit, 2013). Chapter 1 called for educators to remember the needs of the "whole child," and it has been the intention of the revised 2024 SHAPE America National Health Education Standards to not ignore the inequitable conditions or root causes of **health disparities** (e.g., poverty, oppression, structural and institutional racism, discrimination, privilege) and other social determinants of health (SDOH) (see figure 1.1), which affect health functioning and quality-of-life outcomes based on the conditions in which people are born, live, learn, work, play, worship, and age (CDC, 2023; Kendi & Macy, 2023; Benes, 2019; Benes & Alperin, 2022; Office of Disease Prevention and Health Promotion, n.d.). Examples of disproportionate impacts on health outcomes based on race include maternal deaths being three times as high for Black women as they are for white women and the highest among any racial group (Berg, Callaghan, William et al., 2010); fatal injuries among children and adults aged 1 to 44 years old are disproportionately carried by Black and American Indian/Alaska Native (AI/AN) people, as well as those in rural and low-income communities, who are also nearly four times as likely to die from cancer and heart disease (Kendi & Macy, 2023); and even as drowning death rates decrease in recent decades, rates continue to remain high among certain racial/ethnic groups, particularly American Indian/Alaska Native (AI/AN) and Black people (Clemens, et al, 2021).

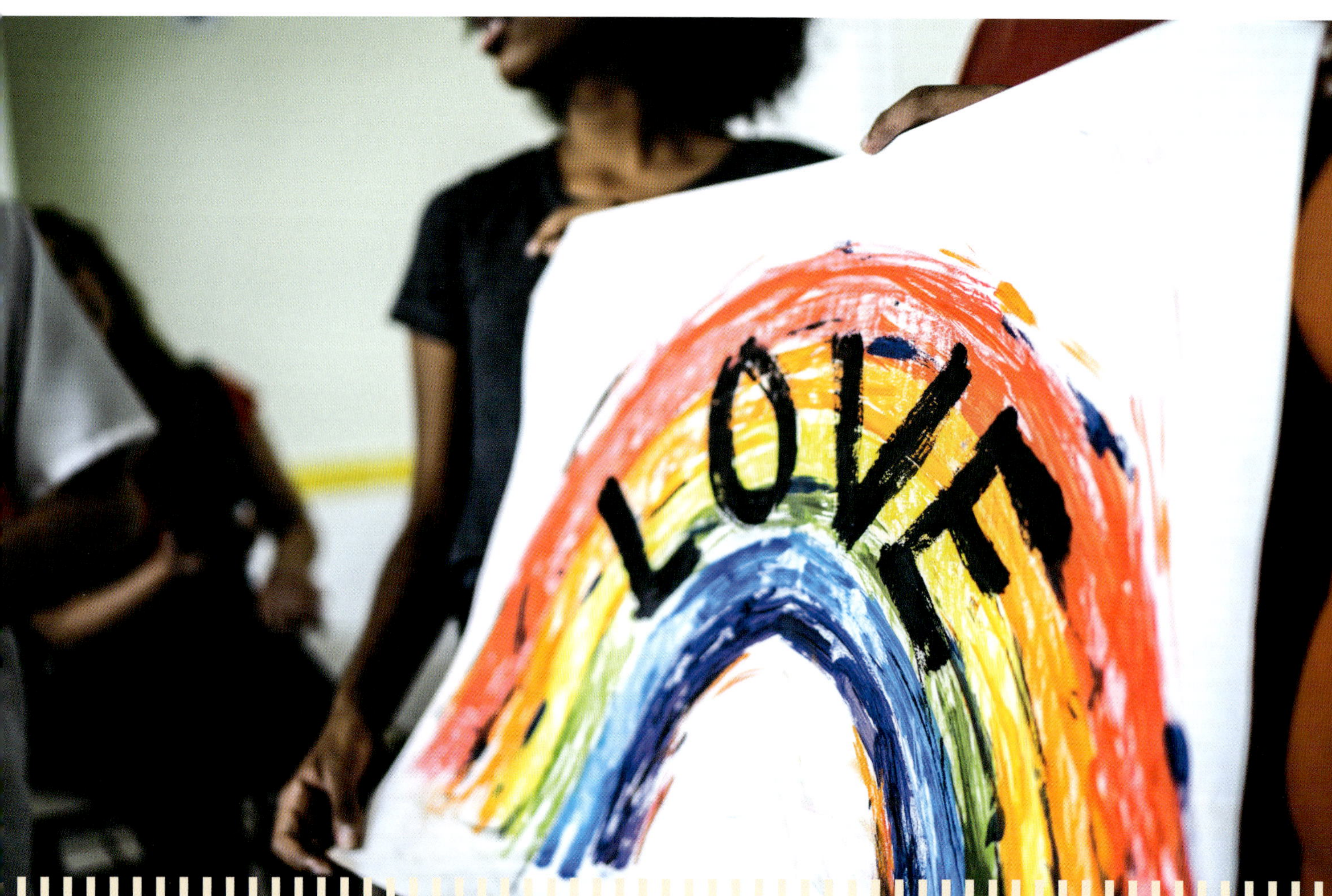

Health Education in Context

School-based preK-12 health education provides the ideal platform for exploring health disparities, power systems, oppression, and social determinants to help students develop critical inquiry and action-oriented skills needed to advance health equity and social justice (Mucedola, 2023; Benes & Alperin, 2022; Benes, 2019). As we strive to reimagine a nation where children and adolescents are health literate, we must recognize that in order to achieve educational equity, and thereby achieve **health equity**, we must apply principles of fairness and justice in the allocation of resources, work toward the elimination of institutional barriers to access, and promote opportunities and positive health outcomes (Kendi & Macy, 2023; Benes, 2019). It is critical that health education be positioned to provide curricular experiences that facilitate students' abilities to evoke the characteristics of **social-emotional learning (SEL)** (e.g., personal and social responsibility, self-awareness, respect, and resilience), which can support their overall learning (CASEL, 2020; Hellison, 2011). For that reason, as health education stakeholders (see chapter 1 description), it is our responsibility to understand, recognize, and contextualize the sociocultural and socioecological perspectives of students and to remove obstacles (i.e., dismantle racist systems and structures, poverty, powerlessness, dehumanization) to help *all* students develop agency, acquire knowledge, and develop the skills needed to lead health-enhancing lives and foster whole-person development (see figure 1.2) (Mucedola, 2023; Killen & Rutland, 2022; Benes & Alperin, 2022; Blackshear & Culp, 2020; Culp, 2021; Benes, 2019; Lovett-Scott & Prather, 2014).

Working for social justice in education means guiding students—and often being guided by students—in critical self-reflection (Cochran-Smith, 2004, as cited by Sensoy & Diangelo, 2009, p. 350; Learning for Justice, n.d.; Benes & Alperin, 2022; Blackshear & Culp, 2020; Benes, 2019). As health educators, our ability to understand the context (i.e., cultural, social, economic, political, geographic, environmental, and demographic) of long-standing issues, historical legacies, and institutional patterns and practices that perpetuate inequality and oppression in our schools and communities is vital (SHAPE America, 2022; Benes, 2019; Benes & Alperin, 2022). Health education can be a part of the solution to "eradicate structural and institutional racism, classism, linguicism, ableism, ageism, heterosexism, religious bias, and xenophobia" (SHAPE America, 2022, p. 6). We must be intentional about demonstrating and modeling critical consciousness, empathy, and respect for each student (Mucedola, 2023; Killen & Rutland, 2022; Benes & Alperin, 2022; SHAPE America, 2022; Beale-Tawfeeq et al., 2018, 2023; Culp, 2021; Blackshear & Culp, 2020; Krawec, 2022; Benes, 2019; Lovett-Scott & Prather, 2014; Munthe, 2008).

A Shared Vision

The Office of Disease Prevention and Health Promotion government report Healthy People 2030 (n.d.) provides a framework and shared vision in which all people and communities can achieve their full potential for health and well-being. It is with this goal in mind that the National Health Education Standards

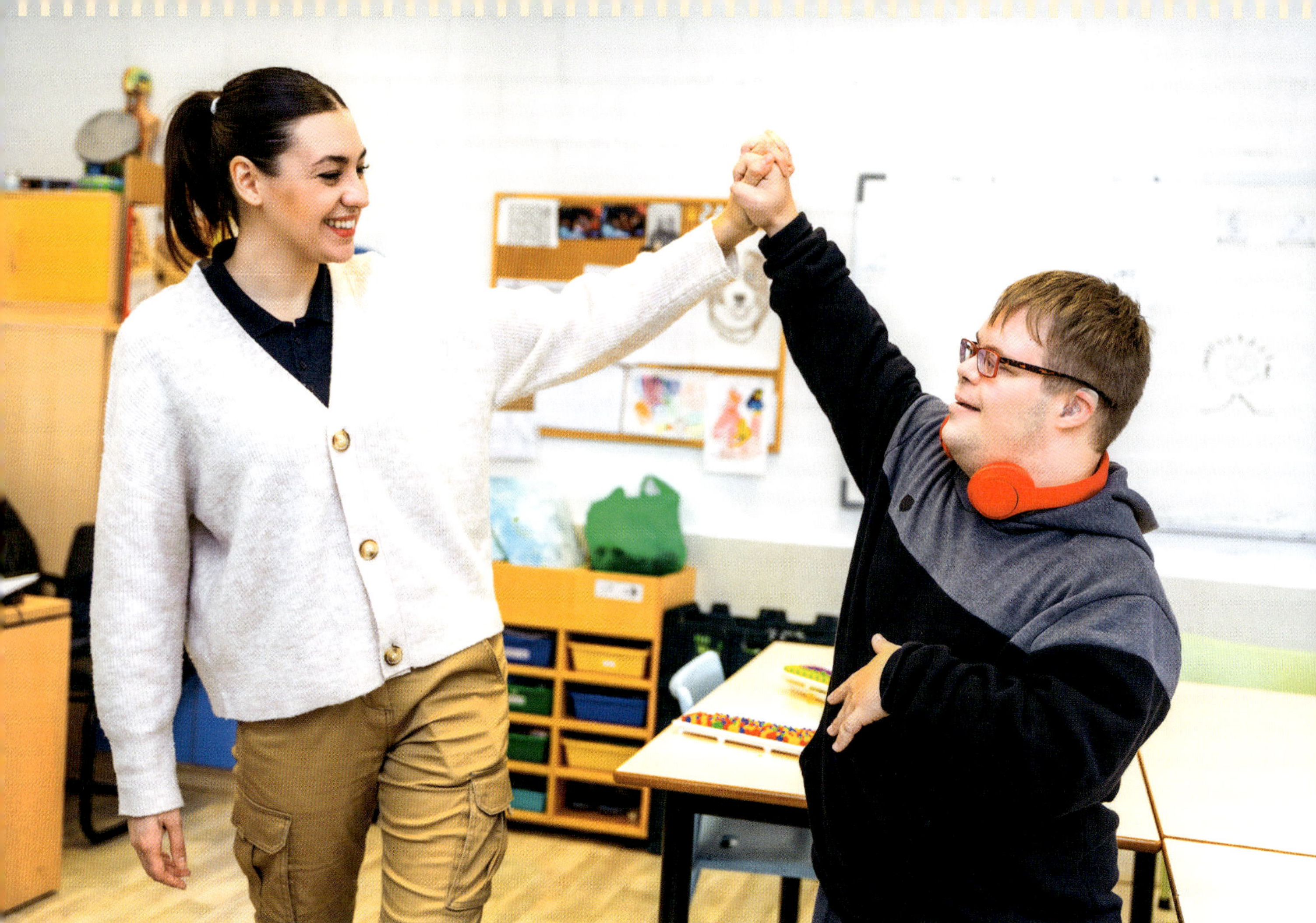

"Education is a universal human right, essential to bridging gaps in human well-being, equity, and opportunity."

Gina Cosentino, Indigenous People Advisory Consultant (2016)

supports health education stakeholders and community of practice (see chapter 1 for stakeholders) in producing school-based health education programs and experiences. These experiences will empower students, families, and communities—regardless of their race, ethnicity, geographic location, economic status, and other SDOH—to become life-saving change agents and health advocates, not only in the classroom but within the context of their everyday lives and communities (Office of Disease Prevention and Health Promotion, n.d.; Kendi & Macy, 2023; SHAPE America, 2022; American Cancer Society, 2007).

Access to equitable, high-quality school-based health education is essential for student attainment of the functional knowledge needed to promote health literacy (see table 3.1; Sensoy & Diangelo, 2009).

Through the collective implementation of the National HE Standards, all students will have access to high-quality health instruction that will increase the awareness of injustices and help students develop the skills needed to make safe, appropriate, healthful choices and minimize health barriers so that everyone can achieve (Benes & Alperin, 2022). True access means that school-based health education should not be sacrificed to other educational or social variables, nor should it be provided in a way that reduces its value. That being the case, as health education stakeholders, we must be willing to create healthy educational learning environments that are integrated within the classroom, curriculum, and community. Even the best standards cannot ensure that all students will learn the

TABLE 3.1 Behavioral Attributes of Health Literacy

Seeking and accessing information	Ability to seek, find, and obtain health information (Bröder et al., 2017, p. 15)
Communication and interaction	Sending and receiving information orally and in written form; understanding and interpreting signals and other cues across a variety of contexts and situations
Application of information	Using health information for health-promoting decisions for self and others
Context-specific skills	Skills such as navigating the health care system, filling out forms, or accessing counseling or other services
Citizenship	The "ability to act in an ethically responsible way and take social responsibility . . . It involves considering health matters beyond one's own perspective, namely through the lens of others and of the collective as well as moving from individual behavior changes toward wider changes" (Bröder et al., 2017, p. 16).

Reprinted by permission from S. Benes and H. Alperin, *The Essentials of Teaching Health Education: Curriculum, Instruction and Assessment*, 2nd ed. (Champaign, IL: Human Kinetics, 2022).

essential concepts and skills embodied in them. However, it is the intent of the National HE Standards to provide a framework of support, and it is understood that every school and community is unique; has diverse capacities and values; and is located in varied cultural, physical, environmental, and social settings. These characteristics demonstrate many of the ways the National HE Standards support the holistic approach of the Whole School, Whole Community, Whole Child (WSCC) model in a school setting. This list is neither final nor complete; rather, it is intended to spark inspiration and dialogue among health educators and health education stakeholders about how to support school-based health education and cultivate healthy schools. Additional action steps can be seen in appendix A.

1. View health education as an academic subject that is a critical part of a well-rounded education
2. Provide health education instructional time and resources equitable to other academic subject areas for preK-12 students
3. Ground instruction in student-centered learning experiences
4. Recognize the importance of the equitable time and resources necessary to accomplish learning and accommodate differences (e.g., environment and climate, teaching, curriculum, assessment, and technology), which are essential to the effective implementation of National HE Standards
5. Demand critical thinking, no matter the methodology or instructional program being used, to ensure that all children and adolescents gain access to basic skills essential to flourish and develop social-emotional skills and strategies that will sustain them whether in the classroom or in life

6. Support students in their development of emotional ego strength to challenge racist societal views of their own competence and worthiness and that of their families and communities
7. Engage in proactive planning that reflects an understanding that every preK-12 school is unique (e.g., student expectations and curricula needs in public school settings differ from suburban schools, and both suburban and inner-city schools differ from rural school settings)
8. Recognize and build on students' strengths and assets, particularly within marginalized communities
9. Recognize the importance of preparing students to be global citizens who will face demographic, technological, and ongoing health care inequity
10. Use familiar metaphors and experiences from the world to connect what students already know to classroom instruction
11. Create a sense of community and caring in the classroom
12. Monitor and assess students' needs and then address them with a wealth of diverse strategies
13. Honor and respect the students' homes and cultures
14. Foster a sense of students' connection to community to something greater than themselves
15. Foster the integration of health and well-being initiatives within all subject areas and not siloed within one curriculum area
16. Foster the inclusion of health, well-being, and holistic elements in a range of school activities (e.g., assemblies, announcements, nutrition breaks, events)
17. Reflect and check to make sure that students and their respective communities can see themselves within the plan

Adapted from Mucedola (2023); Culp (2021); SHAPE America (2022); Benes and Alperin (2022); Canadian Healthy Schools Alliance (2021); Benes (2019); Office of Disease Prevention and Health Promotion (ODPHP) (2018); ESSA (2016); Delpit (2012); Cruz et al. (2011); American Cancer Society (2007); Glasgow, McNary, and Hicks (2006).

Using the National HE Standards to make cross-curricular and interdisciplinary connections allows for a coordinated approach to support school-based health education in meaningful ways among health education stakeholders. By supporting effective school-based health education curricula and programming that is equitable, inclusive, and accessible for all, we can all play a part in creating a healthier nation.

"Health is more than the absence of disease. Health is about jobs and employment, education, the environment, and all of those things that go into making us healthy."

Joycelyn Elders

CHAPTER 4

Developing Curriculum and Instruction

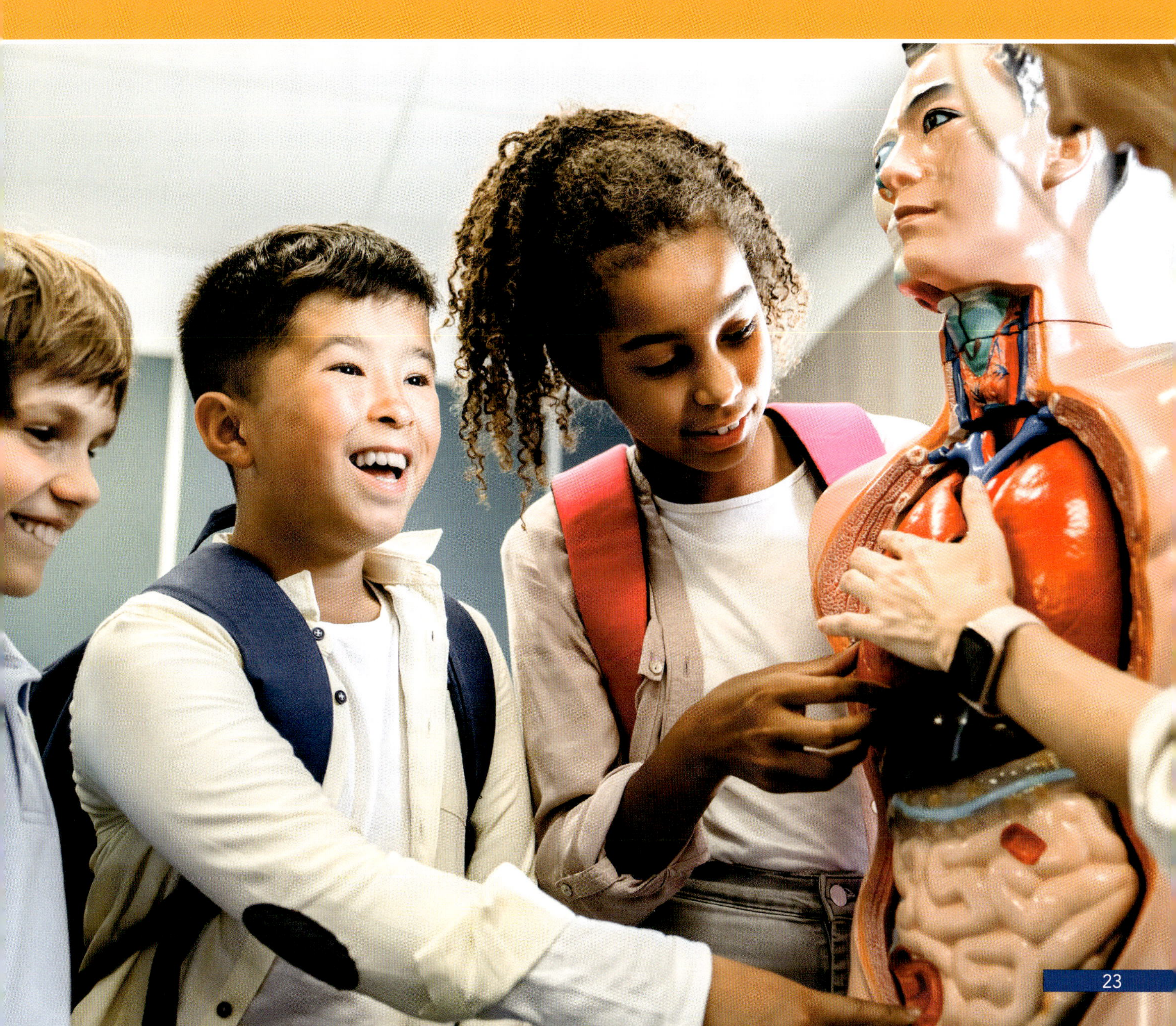

A set of standards describes what students should know and be able to do but is not designed to be **curriculum**. Rather, the 2024 SHAPE America National Health Education Standards serve as a guide during the **curriculum planning** process that ensures that standards, **instructional practices and strategies**, and **assessment** are aligned to promote quality health education (McTighe & Brown, 2020). In this version of the National Health Education Standards, grade span outcomes are framed as performance indicators that include steps for health skill acquisition, and guidance is provided on essential concepts applicable to a variety of health education content areas. Moving forward with the National HE Standards, simply defining which standards are to be taught is not sufficient. By **scaffolding learning**, curriculum materials and resources need to be developed to ensure a logical progression of skills and content within units, across units during the year or course, and from one grade level to the next (Hess, 2023). In order to begin this process, we must start with the standards and performance indicators and work backward to develop curricular and instructional resources (see figure 4.1).

"One looks back with appreciation to the brilliant teachers, but with gratitude to those who touched our human feelings. The curriculum is so much necessary raw material, but warmth is the vital element for the growing plan and for the soul of the child."

Carl Jung

Backward Design

Planning in a standards-based environment is often called *backward design* because it "begins with the end" in mind (Wiggins & McTighe, 2005). In a standards-based classroom, "the end" that teachers concentrate on involves providing evidence of student attainment of the standards and performance indicators (versus completion of a particular activity or project, chapters in a book, or a packaged curriculum). **Authentic assessments**, aligned with standards and performance indicators, are used to provide a clear picture of student learning and measures of instructional effectiveness. Therefore, health teachers are able to use their assessment data as feedback to continually improve the instructional process at every stage.

Backward design is a three-stage approach to designing curriculum by aligning standards, assessment, and instruction (see figure 4.2). The first stage in backward design is to use the standards and performance indicators to identify

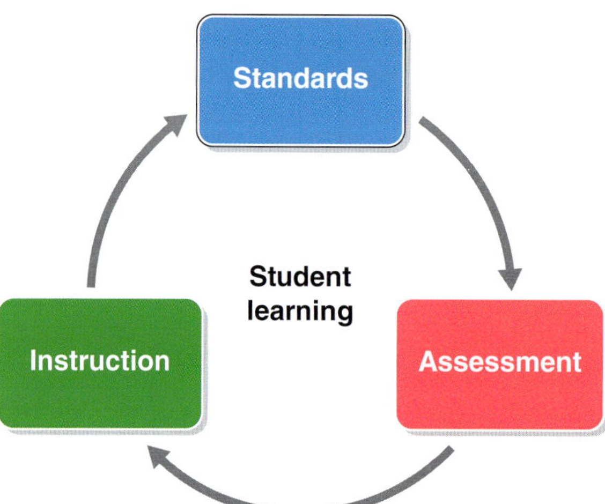

FIGURE 4.1 The link between standards, assessment, and instruction can be thought of as a continuous cycle.

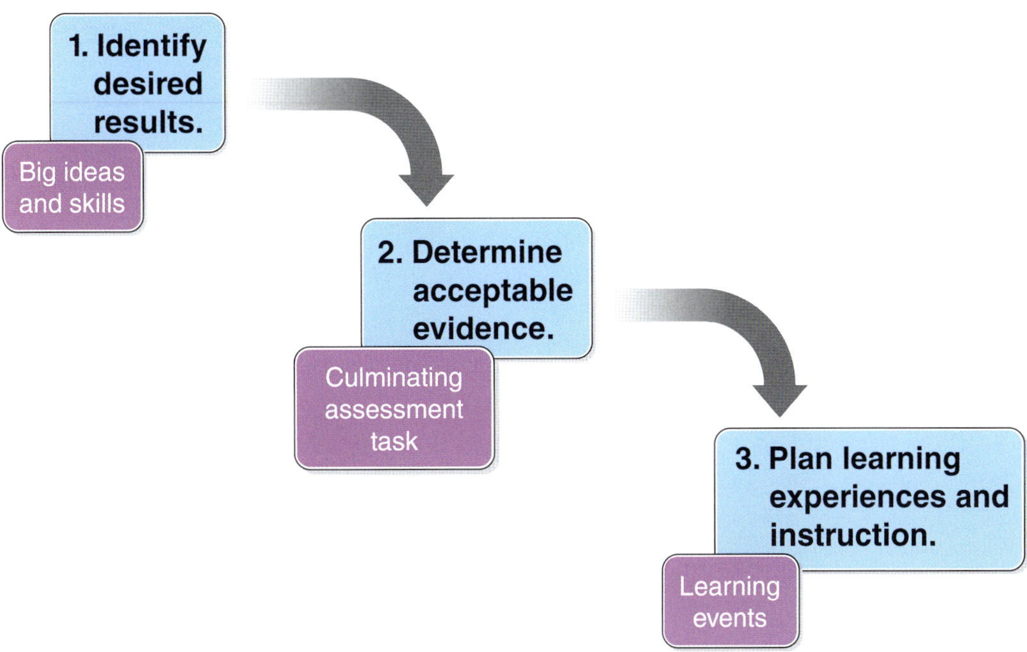

FIGURE 4.2 The backward-design approach to standards-based curriculum and instructional design process. Standards form the foundation for desired results; assessments provide evidence that students are meeting or not meeting the standards, which allows educators to shape curricula and instruction.

Adapted by permission from G. Wiggins and J. McTighe, *Understanding by Design, Expanded*, 2nd ed. (Arlington, VA: ASCD.

the **health-related skills** and concepts that students should know and be able to do. The second stage is to identify assessments that will provide evidence of students' achievement of these skills and concepts. The third stage is to develop the instructional practices that will help students learn and master the identified health-related skills and concepts. Although these three stages outline an approach to the curriculum planning, it is important to understand that these stages are interconnected and that the process is not rigidly linear or step-by-step. Improvements will be made in the development and implementation at each stage in the process.

Curriculum Planning

The first stage of backward design is identifying desired results. This process begins by collecting data related to the skills and concepts currently being taught, the products and performances used to assess students' learning, and community and school health-related data (Carr & Harris, 2001; Jacobs, 2004). The data will guide the selection of standards and performance indicators that are appropriate for the grade level, course, grade span, or preK-12 educational experience. It is often helpful to create a visual representation or a detailed plan, such as a **cur-**

riculum map, that clearly identifies the health skills and concepts that need to be covered to meet the standards as well as district and state requirements (see figure 4.3). Curriculum maps that align with the National HE Standards help educators, administrators, students, and other key stakeholders understand what is expected in the health education curriculum and how progress will be measured.

In this example, Standard 1 is grouped into seven broad functional health information areas aligned with National HE Standards, as well as state and local performance standards and legislative requirements. For each grade level, these broad content areas are paired with one of the seven health skill standards (Standards 2-8).

One important consideration when creating a curriculum map is what health skills and concepts will be covered and the order in which they will be taught, otherwise known as the **scope and sequence**. The scope addresses the breadth and depth of the content and skills that will be covered in the curriculum, while the sequence outlines the order in which they will be taught. At the classroom level, explicit scope and sequence plans ensure that prioritized skills and concepts are covered within the designated time frame. They also assist in planning for appropriate scaffolding of concepts and skills, starting with foundational ideas and gradually moving to more complex concepts, otherwise known as *vertical and horizontal alignment* (see figure 4.4). This alignment helps provide a clear roadmap

Grade	Standard 2: Analyzing Influences	Standard 3: Accessing Information	Standard 4: Interpersonal Communication	Standard 5: Decision-Making	Standard 6: Goal-Setting	Standard 7: Self-Management	Standard 8: Advocacy
Kindergarten	Personal health and wellness	Healthy relationships and family life	Mental and emotional health	Violence prevention	Alcohol, tobacco, and other drugs	Safety	Healthy eating
1st	Mental and emotional health	Violence prevention	Safety	Healthy eating	Personal health and wellness	Alcohol, tobacco, and other drugs	Healthy relationships and family life
2nd	Healthy eating	Safety	Healthy relationships and family life	Personal health and wellness	Mental and emotional health	Violence prevention	Alcohol, tobacco, and other drugs
3rd	Healthy relationships and family life	Alcohol, tobacco, and other drugs	Violence prevention	Safety	Healthy eating	Personal health and wellness	Mental and emotional health
4th	Violence prevention	Mental and emotional health	Alcohol, tobacco, and other drugs	Healthy relationships and family life	Safety	Healthy eating	Personal health and wellness
5th	Alcohol, tobacco, and other drugs	Healthy eating	Personal health and wellness	Safety	Violence prevention	Healthy relationships and family life	Mental and emotional health
6th	Personal health and wellness	Violence prevention	Healthy relationships and family life	Alcohol, tobacco, and other drugs	Healthy eating	Mental and emotional health	Safety
7th	Healthy relationships and family life	Personal health and wellness	Mental and emotional health	Violence prevention	Alcohol, tobacco, and other drugs	Safety	Healthy eating
8th	Mental and emotional health	Safety	Alcohol, tobacco, and other drugs	Personal health and wellness	Healthy relationships and family life	Healthy eating	Violence prevention
High school	Alcohol, tobacco, and other drugs	Personal health and wellness	Violence prevention	Healthy relationships and family life	Healthy eating	Safety	Mental and emotional health

FIGURE 4.3 Sample curriculum map based on the National HE Standards.

for both teachers and students, helping them understand how different topics and skills relate to and build on each other.

Skills-Based Instruction

Curriculum maps and scope and sequence plans using the new National HE Standards may be different than those created in the past since there is an increased emphasis on using both standards and **skills-based instruction** in the curriculum design process. Skills-based curriculum maps involve aligning curriculum components to effectively teach and develop life skills (Benes & Alperin, 2022; Connolly, 2019). Instead of solely providing students with information about health topics, **skills-based health education** places a strong emphasis on equipping students with the skills and strategies they need to lead healthy lives. Therefore, a skills-

Sixth Grade Health Education **Teaching and Learning Framework** **17.00700** **Course description:** Students in sixth grade generate and choose positive alternatives to risky behaviors. They use skills to resist peer pressure and manage stress and anxiety. Students are able to relate health choices (e.g., nutrition, exercise) to alertness, feelings, and performance at school or during physical activity. Students exhibit a healthy lifestyle, interpret health information, and promote good health. Standard 1 is the acquisition of basic health concepts and functional health knowledge and provides a foundation for promoting health-enhancing behaviors among youth. This standard includes essential concepts that are based on established health behavior theories and models. Concepts that focus on both health promotion and risk reduction are included in the performance indicators. This standard is embedded in all health skills and topics. Skills-Based Health Education Resource						
Quarter (9 Weeks)						
Unit 1 1 week	**Unit 2** 1 week	**Unit 3** 2 weeks	**Unit 4** 1 week	**Unit 5** 2 weeks	**Unit 6** 1 week	**Unit 7** 1 week
Semester (18 Weeks)						
Unit 1 3 weeks	**Unit 2** 2 weeks	**Unit 3** 3 weeks	**Unit 4** 2 weeks	**Unit 5** 3 weeks	**Unit 6** 3 weeks	**Unit 7** 2 weeks
Skills Standard 2 Analyzing Influences	**Skills Standard 3** Accessing Information	**Skills Standard 4** Interpersonal Communication	**Skills Standard 5** Decision-Making	**Skills Standard 6** Goal-Setting	**Skills Standard 7** Self-Management	**Skills Standard 8** Advocacy
Topics Personal health Wellness	**Topics** Violence prevention	**Topics** Healthy relationships Family living Disease prevention Sex education AIDS education Growth and development	**Topics** Alcohol Tobacco Other drugs	**Topics** Healthy eating Nutrition	**Topics** Mental health Emotional health Health careers	**Topics** Safety Consumer health Community health Environmental health
Module #'s 11, 12	**Module #'s** 3, 7	**Module #'s** 10, 17, 18	**Module #'s** 13, 14, 15, 16	**Module #'s** 8, 9	**Module #'s** 1, 4, 5, 6	**Module #'s** 19, 20

FIGURE 4.4 This sample scope and sequence is from a school district in Georgia using the curriculum map from figure 4.3. Additional information, such as order, focus areas, and time allocations, is specified on the scope and sequence.

Cobb County School District, Health Education, Sixth Grade Scope and Sequence (2023), Cobb County, Georgia.

based scope and sequence emphasizes the health-related skills and performance indicators included in Standards 2 through 8 while embedding essential health concepts addressed in Standard 1. Instructional units are focused on the health skill and may include one or more health-related content areas (figures 4.3 and 4.4). In order to provide adequate opportunity for students to learn, practice, and attain health-related skills, it may be necessary to reduce the amount of instructional time on health concepts. A skills-based health education curriculum map will emphasize skill development with the inclusion of **functional health information** that will help students develop high levels of health literacy. Functional health information is essential knowledge students must know in order to perform a health skill correctly. Functional health information will vary based on the skill standard in which it is being taught.

Determining Functional Health Information

Determining functional health information is based on student, school, and community data and priorities collected as part of the curriculum-mapping process. Historically, health education curricula were often organized around health content or topic areas. As health education has shifted to a more standards- and skills-based approach, many states, districts, and schools use local and school data to determine health priority areas (see figure 4.4). When local data are not available, the Centers for Disease Control and Prevention has identified nine health content areas to address adolescent health priorities (see figure 4.5; Centers for Disease Control and Prevention, 2021). This list is not exhaustive, and data may support a more holistic approach that includes topical areas traditionally included in a **comprehensive school health education** program. The National HE Standards provide a framework from which curricula can be developed based on the identified priority areas to ensure health content and concepts are tailored to local needs. This approach allows the National HE Standards to remain relevant over time, despite changing data on health priorities. It also allows the National HE Standards to serve as a national framework that can be customized to address the state and local health needs of students. Once the health content areas are determined, it is still important to clarify what health information needs to be included in the instructional materials.

Many state and local agencies will use the National HE Standards to provide further direction to local educational agencies to assist them with development of specific curricula that meet national and state standards. In recognition of this process, the National HE Standards do not address specific health education content areas explicitly. Instead, they provide a framework from which curricula can be developed, allowing for the inclusion of functional health information that is appropriate for local needs (see table 4.1).

Common health education content areas	*National Health Education Standards, Third Edition*	Centers for Disease Control and Prevention Health Education Curriculum Analysis Tool modules
• Personal and community health • Nutrition • Physical activity • Growth, development, and sexual health • Injury prevention and safety • Mental, emotional, and social health • Alcohol and other drugs • Tobacco • Media and digital health literacy • Chronic and communicable disease prevention • Environmental health • Consumer health	**Standard 1** Use functional health information to support health and well-being of self and others. **Standard 2** Analyze influences that affect health and well-being of self and others. **Standard 3** Access valid and reliable resources to support health and well-being of self and others. **Standard 4** Use interpersonal communication skills to support health and well-being of self and others. **Standard 5** Use a decision-making process to support health and well-being of self and others. **Standard 6** Use a goal-setting process to support health and well-being of self and others. **Standard 7** Demonstrate practices and behaviors to support health and well-being of self and others. **Standard 8** Advocate to promote health and well-being of self and others.	• Personal health and wellness • Food and nutrition • Physical activity • Sexual health • Safety • Mental and emotional health • Alcohol and other drugs • Tobacco • Violence prevention

FIGURE 4.5 The interrelationship of common health education content areas, the National HE Standards, and the Centers for Disease Control and Prevention's Health Education Curriculum Analysis Tool (HECAT) modules. The standards are designed to encompass a wide range of content areas based on local and school data.

TABLE 4.1 Examples of Matching Health Content to Performance Indicators

CONTENT: PREVENTING THE SPREAD OF DISEASE	
GRADES PREK-2	
Performance indicator	**Infused performance indicators**
1.2.3 Identify ways to prevent or reduce risks for illnesses and injuries.	1.2.3 Identify ways to prevent or reduce risks for illnesses and injuries, such as washing hands. • *Assessment:* Identify one way that handwashing removes germs from the hands. • *Instruction:* How washing hands removes germs from the hands.
7.2.2 Demonstrate practices and behaviors that support health and well-being of self and others.	7.2.2 Demonstrate practices and behaviors that support health and well-being of self and others, such as demonstrating the steps of handwashing. • *Assessment:* Correctly demonstrate the steps of handwashing. • *Instruction:* Explain and demonstrate proper steps of handwashing followed by student practice. Pairing performance indicator 1.2.3 with 7.2.2 provides the teacher with the content of why it is important to wash hands, and students practice of the skill of handwashing.
CONTENT: IMPORTANCE OF HAVING POSITIVE FRIENDS WHEN BEING BULLIED	
GRADES 3-5	
Performance indicator	**Infused performance indicators**
1.5.2 Describe health-promoting behaviors for the dimensions of wellness.	1.5.2 Describe health-promoting behaviors for the dimensions of wellness, such as the importance of having healthy friendships. • *Assessment:* Describe two ways having healthy friendships affects each dimension of wellness. • *Instruction:* Describe each dimension of wellness and how healthy relationships affect each dimension of wellness.
2.5.1 Explain how various influences affect health and well-being.	2.5.1 Explain how various influences affect health and well-being when being bullied. • *Assessment:* Explain two ways being bullied affects health and well-being (dimensions of health). • *Instruction:* Define types of bullying, effects of bullying on health and well-being (dimensions of health), benefits of having positive friends when being bullied, and how healthy friends help each other cope when being bullied. Pairing performance indicator 1.5.2 with 2.5.1 provides the teacher with the content of healthy friendships, and students practice the skill of analyzing the influence of bullying on health and well-being and how healthy friends help each other cope when being bullied.

CONTENT: VAPING

GRADES 6-8	
Performance indicator	**Infused performance indicators**
1.8.5 Analyze the connections between health literacy and health outcomes.	1.8.5 Analyze the connections between health literacy and health outcomes regarding vaping. • *Assessment:* Analyze three facts about vaping, three facts about how vaping affects the body, and three ways to use the information to improve well-being. • *Instruction:* Define health literacy, analyze how vaping affects the body, and explain how to use the information to improve well-being.
3.8.5 Use strategies to manage misinformation and disinformation.	3.8.5 Use strategies to manage misinformation and disinformation about vaping. • *Assessment:* Examine the validity and reliability of four vaping websites (two valid and reliable sites and two sites that are not valid or reliable); write down two examples of misinformation about vaping, two examples of disinformation about vaping, and four examples of valid and reliable information about vaping. • *Instruction:* Describe how to determine the validity of website information, how to identify misinformation and disinformation, how to access websites with accurate information about vaping, and how to inform peers of misinformation and disinformation about vaping. Pairing performance indicator 1.8.5 with 3.8.5 provides the teacher with the tools to analyze how to be health literate about vaping, how to access valid and reliable information about vaping, and ways to correct misinformation and disinformation about vaping.

CONTENT: TEXTING AND DRIVING

GRADES 9-12	
Performance indicator	**Infused performance indicators**
1.12.7 Analyze the benefits of and barriers to practicing a variety of health behaviors.	1.12.7 Analyze the benefits of and barriers to practicing a variety of health behaviors, such as not texting while driving. • *Assessment:* Analyze three benefits of and three barriers to not texting while driving. • *Instruction:* Define *benefit and barrier,* and explain the dangers of texting while driving.
8.12.2 Advocate for health issues either collaboratively or individually to promote health and well-being.	8.12.2 Advocate for health issues, such as not texting while driving, either collaboratively or individually to promote health and well-being. • *Assessment:* Design three public service announcements (PSA), collaboratively or individually, that advocate for teens to not text and drive. • *Instruction:* Define *advocacy*, and explain how to design a PSA, directed to teens, about not texting and driving. Pairing performance indicator 1.12.7 with 8.12.2 provides the teacher with the opportunity to challenge teens about the benefits of, and barriers to, not texting while driving and then uses that information to design PSA.

Identifying Assessments

The second stage of backward design is identifying assessments that provide evidence of the standards and performance indicators identified during the curriculum planning process. Effective assessment practices are outlined more fully in chapter 5; however, it is important to note here that assessments must be well thought out and designed prior to the development of instructional materials. Activities and projects used previously in the health classroom may need to be revised or discarded so that assessments will align with the National HE Standards and identified outcomes. In addition, in order to authentically assess student learning, particularly when measuring health skill attainment, assessments need to provide opportunities for students to demonstrate their learning of both health skills and concepts (Benes & Alperin, 2022). Traditional assessment measures, such as tests and quizzes, measure knowledge acquisition but provide limited opportunity for students to demonstrate proficiency in skill development of Standards 2 through 8. The use of **performance-based assessments** is encouraged so that students can demonstrate their learning in authentic ways.

Creating Learning Plans

In the third stage of backward design, the methods and materials used for teaching health-related skills and concepts are chosen or created now that teachers, administrators, and other school personnel have established the tasks that students must complete to demonstrate their knowledge and skills. This requires careful consideration of the extent to which instructional units and lesson plans are effective, engaging, and focused around student learning experiences that engage students in health skill building and acquisition of functional health information. This process may involve eliminating content and activities that are not aligned with National HE Standards. To ensure alignment, learning plans should provide opportunities for students to learn the steps or cues for performing the health skills, see examples of skills being used in real-life, have opportunities to practice skills in realistic situations, and receive appropriate feedback from peers and teachers (see figure 4.6). **Student engagement** in the learning process is key to building student self-efficacy to apply their learning in authentic real-world settings.

Health teachers should not be expected to redesign instructional materials in isolation. Working together with other health teachers, as well as district leaders and curriculum experts, is essential for implementation of the National HE Standards. Those working to develop new resource materials, instructional units, and curricula based on the National HE Standards need expertise in health education, assessment design, diversity and equity, inclusive and developmentally appropriate practices, and health pedagogy (Penuel et al., 2011). The time spent by these professionals in the backward design process increases the likelihood that the resulting materials support effective teaching and learning practices needed for students to achieve higher levels of understanding and skill proficiency. In addition, the process supports **differentiated instruction** and individualized instruction by identifying opportunities to tailor the learning experiences based on students' needs (Tomlinson, 2016).

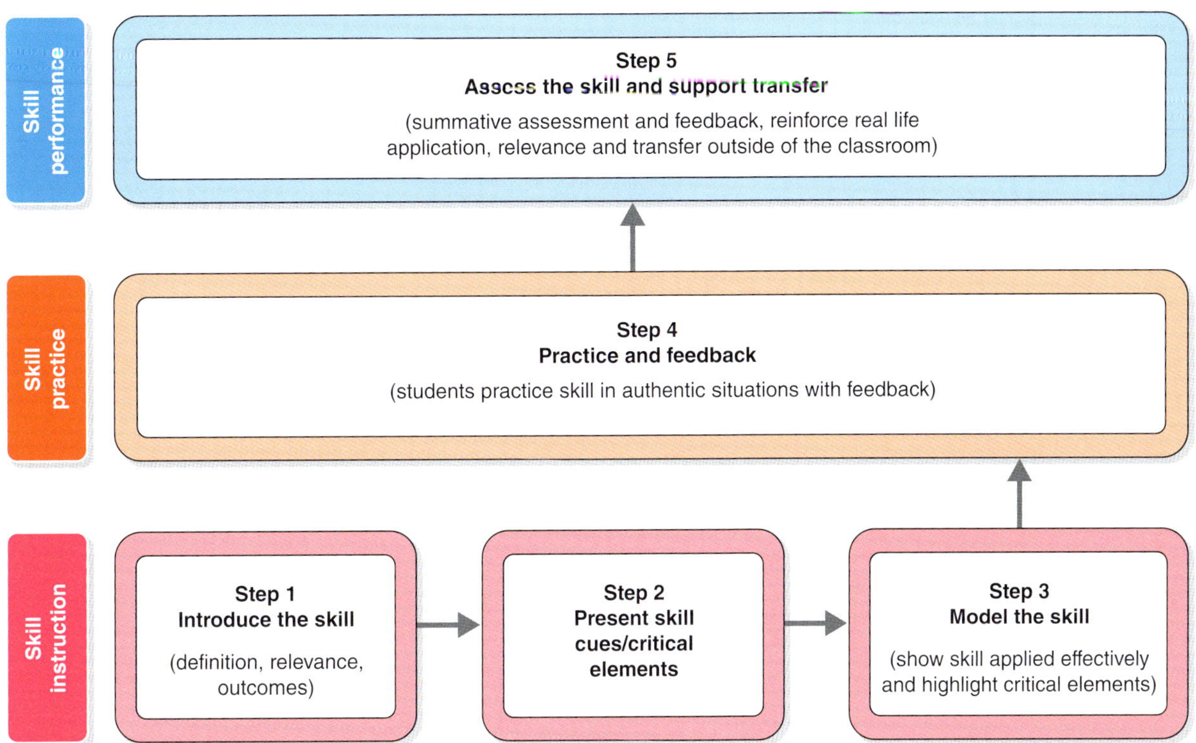

FIGURE 4.6 The skill development model informs the creation of instructional units and lesson plans by setting the stage for skill exploration, practice, and assessment.

Reprinted by permission from S. Benes and H. Alperin, *The Essentials of Teaching Health Education: Curriculum, Instruction and Assessment*, 2nd ed. (Champaign, IL: Human Kinetics, 2022).

While the National HE Standards do support both a standards- and skills-based approach to health education, they do not dictate a single approach to instruction. Teachers can organize a variety of activities and experiences in their classroom that promote student learning aligned with National HE Standards. The scope and sequence of these activities will be guided by a curriculum map and supported by curriculum resources that are well matched to that plan. Classroom instruction should be carried out by licensed health education teachers with disciplinary expertise to consistently make decisions about what best meets their students' learning needs.

Universal Design for Learning

Universal design for learning (UDL) is an approach used to maximize the learning of all students (see figure 4.7). Universal design is the creation of instructional resources and assessments that are usable by all students, to the greatest extent feasible, without the need for accommodations and adaptations. Universal design upholds three core principles: representation, engagement, and expression. Representation encourages educators to present information and content in a variety of formats to address different **learning styles** and preferences. Using visual, auditory, multimedia, and kinesthetic materials to teach a new concept

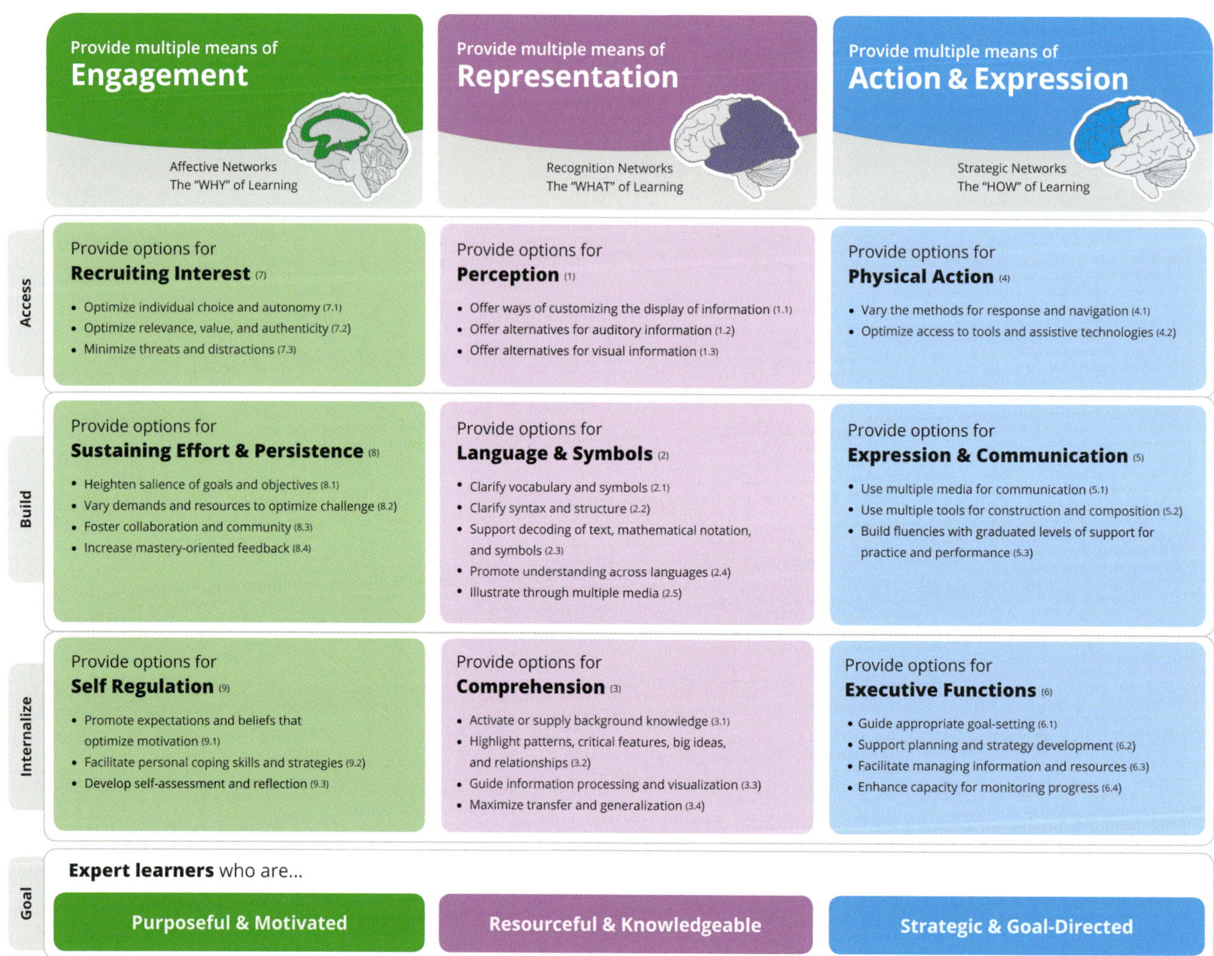

FIGURE 4.7 The universal design for learning model.

© CAST, Inc., 2018. Universal Design for Learning Guidelines Version 2.2 (graphic organizer) Wakefield, MA: Author.

or skill is an example of representation. Offering diverse ways for students to engage in learning, such as experiential learning, real-world applications, and varied instructional strategies, helps address students' different interests and levels of engagement. The principle of expression encourages educators to provide students with a variety of options and opportunities to demonstrate their understanding. This might include offering students options for assignments, presentations, multimedia projects, or other forms of assessment that align with their preferred learning style.

Instructional Practices

In order to fully engage students in the health classroom, the structure of classroom activities and discussions may need to evolve to include more **participatory teaching activities** (Benes & Alperin, 2022; Connolly, 2019). Health teachers build instructional plans that allow them to guide student learning and practice of skills and concepts outlined by National HE Standards. They create a classroom environment that builds trust and rapport between the teacher and the students and among students. Teachers guide and facilitate student learning while students practice application of skills and concepts. Throughout the class, health educators provide opportunities for students to apply new learnings and reflect on their significance in the students' own lives. SHAPE America's *Appropriate Practices for School-Based Health Education* provides an overview of what instruction developed or adapted to support the National HE Standards might resemble and some changes that may be required in the classroom to move forward (SHAPE America, 2015). Instructional practices that reflect the *Characteristics of Effective Health Education* (CDC, 2019) and foster alignment with National HE Standards provide opportunities for the health teacher to do the following:

- Deliver instruction that is guided by, and focused on, the achievement of learning objectives
- Use formative assessment to monitor progress toward objectives
- Deliver instruction that facilitates skill development leading to proficiency
- Employ instructional strategies that promote student self-reflection and help students personalize the lesson
- Implement activities and use materials that are current, up to date, and relevant to students
- Implement participatory teaching and cooperative learning styles
- Engage families and the community in the learning process
- Differentiate instruction to meet the needs of all learners
- Use different modes of delivery and a variety of approaches to engage all students and meet the needs of all learners
- Adjust instruction during lessons, as necessary, to meet the needs of all learners
- Demonstrate passion and enthusiasm for health education

It may take time for schools and health teachers to transition their curricular and instructional practices to a more standards- and skills-based approach. Some are further along with this process than others, having already been aligned with previous versions of the National HE Standards. Health teachers will likely need ongoing support to move toward a standards-based approach that fully integrates skills-based health instruction. As new curriculum materials are developed and adopted or evidence-based curricula is selected, health educators need professional development and collaboration to ensure effective use of these new health resources.

CHAPTER 5

Assessment

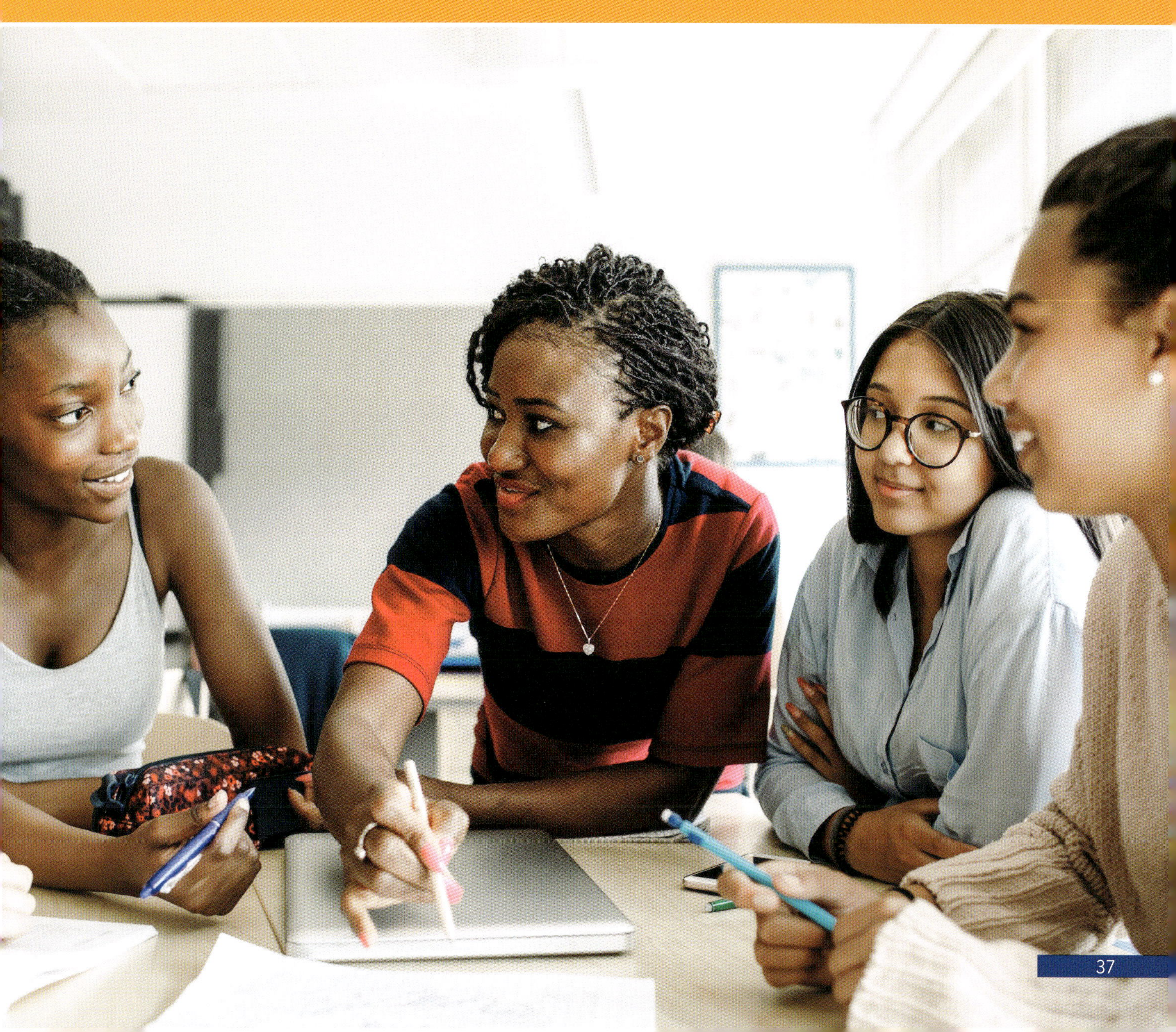

Assessment (stage 2) is an integral part of backward design (see figure 4.2). It provides the evidence to determine student acquisition of health content and skills (stage 1) and serves as a guide to planning the learning experiences and instruction (stage 3). Student attainment of content and skills contributes to the development of behavior that supports health and well-being.

The standards and performance indicators generate assessment and instruction and are explained at the beginning of a unit. Assessment is continuous and includes using targeted feedback and a variety of assessment and instructional strategies to help the student acquire the established goals (standards) and objectives (performance indicators) (Centers for Disease Control and Prevention, 2021).

"If it is worth teaching, it is worth assessing."

CCSSO-SCASS Health Education Assessment Project (2006)

Purpose of Assessment

The purpose of assessment is to "increase student achievement" (Saphier et al., 2017, p. 549). To determine if the student has achieved and is able to demonstrate the performance indicators, the teacher gathers evidence of student learning from a variety of formative assessments. The evidence may indicate that the student has achieved the requirements of the performance indicator, that the teacher needs to reteach using different words and strategies, or that the student needs more time to process the information, to access help, and to complete the assignments.

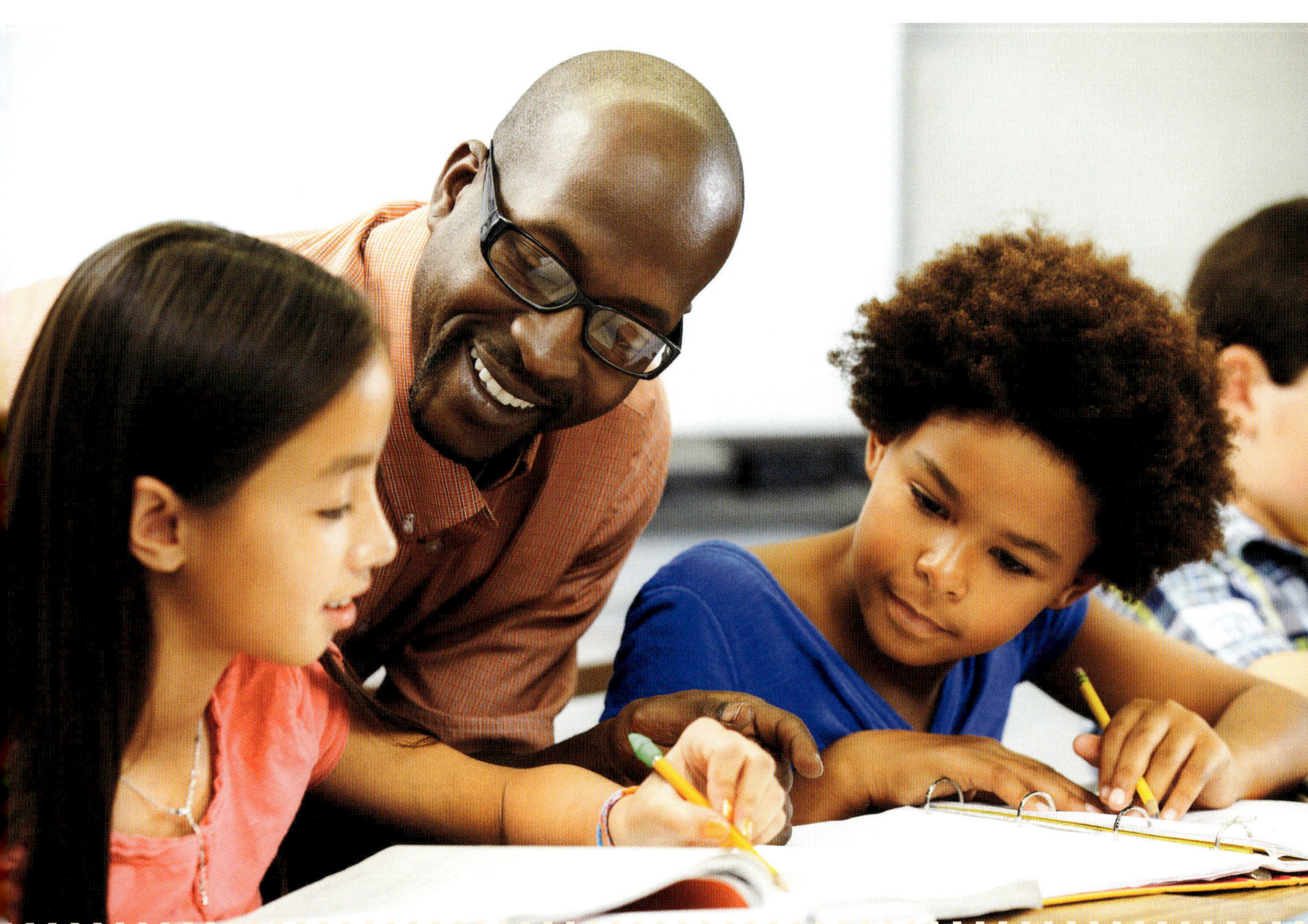

The Assessment Cycle

Backward design, in which assessment is the second step, is the linear process of designing curriculum (see chapter 4). The **assessment cycle** is another way to think about standards, assessment, and instruction (see figure 5.1).

To assess student learning, start by establishing clear, measurable objectives or outcomes by selecting a Standard 1 (content) performance indicator and pairing it with a skill performance indicator from Standards 2 through 8.

Teach the content and the skill, then allow time for student practice. While students are practicing, formatively assess and provide effective feedback. Based on the information learned, reteach, allow additional time, or continue instruction.

Teachers plan and deliver instruction that includes a variety of learning strategies that contribute to student acquisition of health content and skills. Assessment,

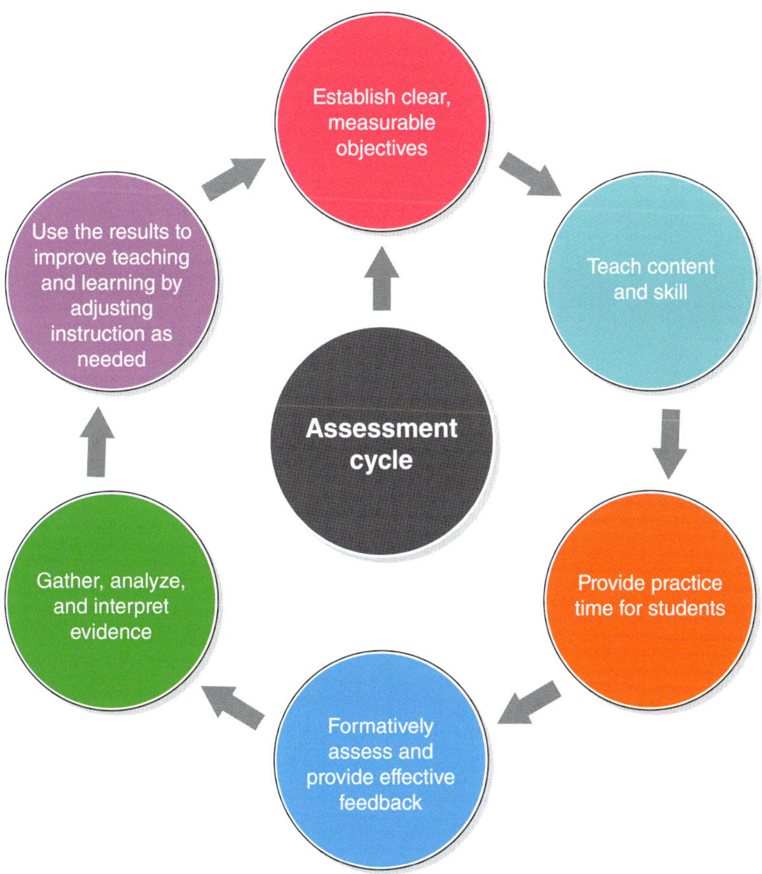

FIGURE 5.1 The assessment cycle.

Reprinted by permission from M. Connolly *Skills-Based Health Education*, 2nd ed. (Burlington, MA: Jones & Bartlett Learning, 2020), 74. www.jblearning.com.

whether it is formative or summative, provides evidence of student learning resulting from these efforts. The summative evidence is reported as a grade to inform the school administration, parents or guardians, district administrators, school committees, and so forth of student progress (Centers for Disease Control and Prevention, 2021).

When beginning a unit, teachers explain the objectives, performance indicators, additional standards (e.g., sex education standards), and daily formative and end-of-unit summative assessments. Knowing how they are being assessed helps students stay focused on reaching the unit objectives. When it is time to begin the summative performance assessment, teachers distribute the **prompts**, backup materials, self-checks, rubrics, and other documents that provide directions and support and help the students achieve the learning goals.

Using this strategy, students have the information they need to take responsibility for their learning, and teachers are prepared to make improvements to instruction if needed (Centers for Disease Control and Prevention, 2021).

Feedback

How do educators help students achieve the content and skill stated in the performance indicators? They make the standards-based learning goals clear, teach the content and skill, formatively assess, and provide opportunities for the students to practice and meet the goals. Students may need additional time for review, to revise their work, to improve, and to learn from their mistakes.

For students to improve, the teacher provides feedback and acknowledges student strengths, celebrates their progress, and reflects on how to continue their content and skill development.

"Everyone—students and teachers—learns through clearly identifying objectives and then using feedback to improve understanding of those objectives."

Myron Dueck (2022)

Using self-checks and providing frequent formative assessment accompanied by effective **feedback** enhances student achievement of the learning goals. Feedback is effective when it compares the student evidence to lesson objectives. For example, if the objective of the lesson is to learn and to be able to demonstrate refusal skills and the teacher responds, "Good job," then the student feels good but does not know why. If the teacher says, "Good job! You have demonstrated each of the four refusal steps accurately and with confidence," then the student knows why he or she did a good job.

Another key to effective feedback is the relationship between the student and the teacher. How the student interprets and receives the feedback and acts on the suggestions is directly related to their relationship. In the scenario above, imagine the student does not demonstrate all the refusal steps and does not speak with confidence.

If the student and the teacher do not have a positive relationship, the student may become discouraged, give up, or dismiss the feedback. If the student and the teacher have a positive relationship such that the teacher delivers the feedback in a caring way that promotes and reinforces their relationship, the student is more open to listening and making the appropriate changes to improve (Frey, 2022).

Consider the following criteria for effective feedback:

- *Growth oriented*: The focus is on strengths, assets, and growth.
- *Real*: Feedback targets the performance indicators and provides specific things the student can do to improve content and skill performance.

- *Empathetic:* Understanding how a student may receive the feedback is key to the student's accepting the feedback. A positive teacher/student relationship enhances the student's acceptance of feedback.
- *Asked for:* While providing feedback, the teacher encourages the student to ask questions and seek additional feedback.
- *Timely:* To be most effective, feedback is frequent and provided soon after the formative assessment (Frey, 2022).
- *Understandable:* The feedback informs the student of what was done well, what needs improvement, and how to make the improvements (McTighe, 2005).

Backward Design

The backward design model is explained in chapter 4 and reviewed earlier in this chapter. In figure 5.2, data collection and analysis is added to the model to provide direction to the selection of standards and performance indicators.

When deciding what and how to assess, the following factors should be considered.

1. Start by reviewing national, state, or local data that document the health of youth.
2. Select a Standard 1 (content) performance indicator and pair it with a skill performance indicator from Standards 2 through 8 to reduce risk behaviors and enhance student health and well-being.
3. When planning the assessment, ask, "What do I want the students to do to demonstrate that they are proficient in the performance indicators?" Use the verbs from the performance indicators to inform the assessment.
   - If the verb is to *analyze*, the student provides evidence of the ability to analyze. A graphic organizer is an effective tool to use to help students analyze (see figure 5.3).
   - *Demonstrate* is a common skills verb. In this case, students show the teacher what they have learned. For example, students demonstrate refusal skills, goal-setting skills, decision-making skills, and so on.
4. Once the assessment is determined for the content and skill, plan the instruction. Ask, "What do I need to teach to help my students be successful on the assessment?"

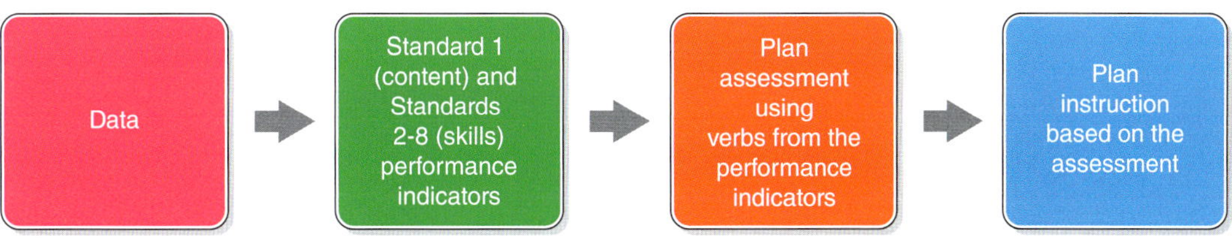

FIGURE 5.2 Backward design, including data collection and analysis.

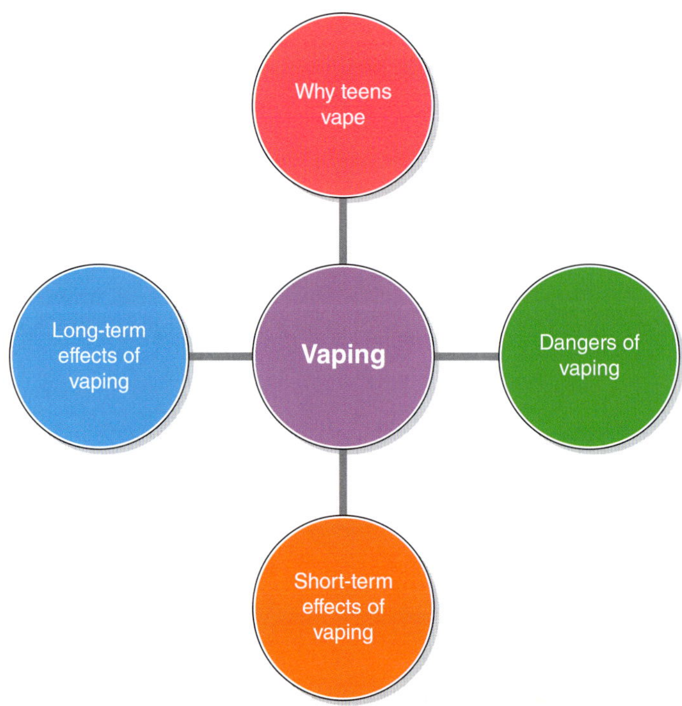

FIGURE 5.3 Graphic organizer.

Formative Assessment

Formative assessment is assessment *for* learning (see figure 5.4). In order for learning to take place, the students must understand the objectives of the unit or lesson and how they are going to reach them. The objectives in the skills-based classroom are the content and skill performance indicators.

At the beginning of a unit, teachers help students identify what they already know and preview the learning by giving a preassessment or an inventory of upcoming instruction. Other options include completing a What I Know, What I Want to Know, and What I Learned (KWL) chart, a concept map, and participating in classroom discussion (Brookhart, 2024).

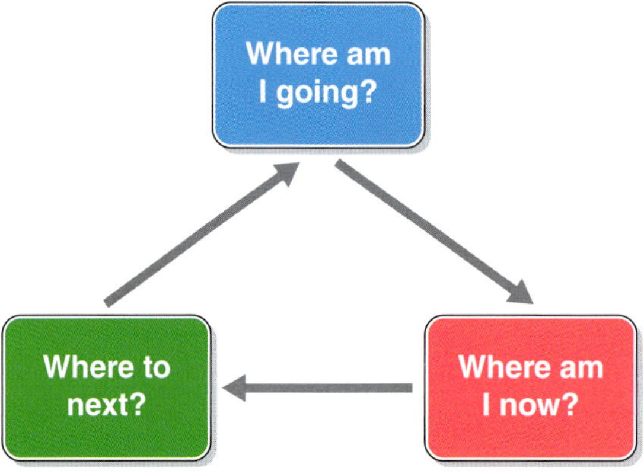

FIGURE 5.4 Formative assessment learning cycle.

Adapted by permission from S.M. Brookhart and J. McTighe, *The Formative Assessment Learning Cycle (Quick Reference Guide)* (Arlington, VA: ASCD. © 2005). All rights reserved.

As instruction begins, frequent formative assessment helps gauge student acquisition of content and skill performance indicators. It also provides the teacher with the opportunity to provide effective feedback and coach the students to meet the learning objectives. An analysis of the formative assessments provides valuable information to the teacher, who then must decide whether to continue instruction, pause to clarify instruction, or stop to reteach.

Weaving formative assessment throughout instruction provides students with the opportunity to improve content and skill acquisition over time and contributes to achieving the performance indicators of the summative assessment.

Districts transform their assessment strategies when they use formative assessment to help teachers adjust their instruction to meet the needs of the students rather than focusing on the collection of grades to compare student achievement (Popham, 2008).

Types of Formative Assessments

Many types of formative assessments can be employed. Some formative assessments are used during face-to-face instruction, and other formative assessments are designed for online use. Regardless of the differences between these types, each provides the teacher with information about the progress of student learning and the opportunity to reteach or provide additional practice time if necessary.

Examples of formative assessments include those found in table 5.1.

A variety of electronic interactive applications exist to help students and teachers engage and provide evidence of student learning. Following are a few examples:

- *Near Pod:* Provides the infrastructure to create interactive lessons, videos, activities, and formative assessments (Near Pod, 2023).
- *Lumio:* A digital learning tool that engages students. It is designed to provide collaborative learning experiences, including formative assessment (Lumio, 2023).
- *Microsoft Flip:* A free app that provides students with the ability to express their ideas asynchronously in video, text, and audio messages (Microsoft, 2023).
- *Mentimeter:* An interactive platform that provides the opportunity to test knowledge, gather opinions, start discussions, and so on (Mentimeter, 2023).
- *Mural:* An interactive digital whiteboard that provides the opportunity to work together on projects, gather opinions, and so forth (Mural, 2023).

Because skills-based health is student-centered and engaging and encourages continuous acquisition of the content and skills performance indicators, students have the opportunity to revise their work to better meet the standards. This strategy uses the results of formative assessments and aligns the student and the teacher with the goal of continuous improvement rather than a particular grade.

TABLE 5.1 Formative Assessments

Formative	Use
Bow tie	The topic or challenge is placed on the knot. Students place responses on the bow. *Example:* The topic is eating breakfast every day. On the left side of the bow, the student writes down three benefits of eating breakfast every day. On the right side of the bow, the student writes down three barriers to eating breakfast every day.
Continuums	The continuum provides individual information when used by one student and provides group information when used by a team. *Example:* Place a check mark on the arrow to show your progress completing a SMART goal.
Sorts	Sorts work well with content or skills that have a sequence of steps, such as handwashing. *Example:* • Write or draw the steps of handwashing. • Cut the steps into strips. • Place the strips in a baggie and distribute among students. • Students draw the strips and place them in order. A self-check is available to review accuracy.
Sticky notes	Sticky notes can be used in a variety of ways to collect students' responses. *Examples:* • Exit tickets: Students write their response to an exit ticket and place their sticky note by the door as they leave. The teacher reviews student answers. • Sticky splash: The teacher writes a question on the board. Students respond on a sticky note and place their response on the board. The teacher reviews student answers. • Venn diagram: The teacher draws a Venn diagram on the board and labels one circle "Pro" and the other circle "Con." The teacher asks a question and students write a pro or con statement on a sticky note. Students place their sticky note on the Venn diagram. The teacher reviews student answers.
Targets	Targets are used in individual or group formative assessment. The teacher asks for a progress check, and the students place a check on the target that reflects their progress on an activity or project or their understanding of a concept (Connolly, 2020). *Examples:* • Individual: The target might be labeled as "I've got it," "I'm almost there," and "I'm not sure." Students decide which target to check. As the teacher walks around the classroom, he or she sees the students' responses and uses that information to discuss the project. • Group: The target might be labeled as "we've got it", "we're almost there," and "we're not sure." Each group decides which target to check. As the teacher walks around the classroom, he or she sees the groups' responses and uses that information to discuss the project.

<table>
<tr>
<td>Traffic-signal technique
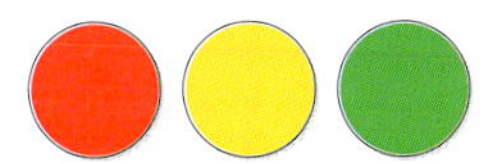</td>
<td>Circles can be used in a variety of ways.
Examples:
• The teacher asks about student readiness. Students hold up their green (ready), yellow (need more time), or red (not ready) circle.
• The teacher poses a question in the form of true or false. Students raise their green (true), yellow (not sure), or red (false) circle.</td>
</tr>
<tr>
<td>Letter card responses
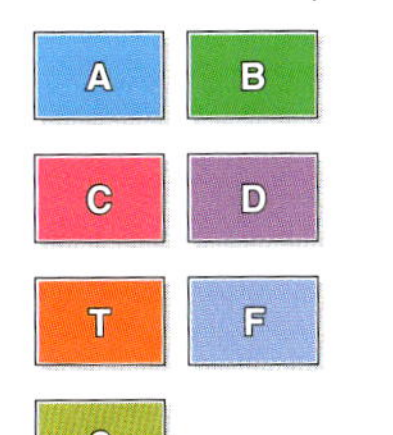
</td>
<td>Letter card responses are used to review or preview information or knowledge of skills. Students have a packet of index cards labeled A, B, C, D, T, F, ?
Examples
• Multiple-choice: The teacher poses a question and reads a list of answer choices labeled A, B, C, D. Students hold up the letter card they think represents the correct answer.
• True/false: The teacher reads a statement in the form of true or false. Students raise their T, F, or ? card.</td>
</tr>
<tr>
<td>Whiteboards
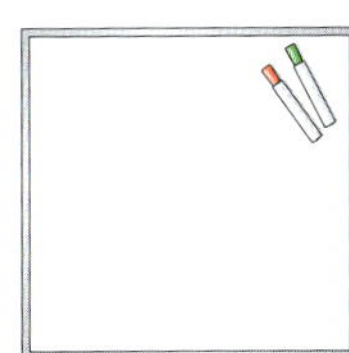</td>
<td>Whiteboards are used individually or by a group. Whiteboards help the teacher quickly assess student progress (Popham, 2008).
Examples
• The teacher asks a question. Students draw or state their response on their whiteboards.
• Students take notes on their whiteboards in preparation for their authentic assessment.
• The teacher asks a preview, review, or reinforcement question. Groups respond on their whiteboards.</td>
</tr>
<tr>
<td colspan="2">Additional examples of formative assessments include hand signals, open-ended questions, quick writes, question box, KWL chart, and concept maps (Brookhart, 2024).</td>
</tr>
</table>

Summative Assessment

Summative assessment is assessment *of* learning. There are a variety of summative assessments, but in skills-based health education the authentic performance assessment, the performance task, is preferred. The performance task provides the evidence needed to determine if students learned the content and are able to perform the skill.

The performance task includes a real-world, engaging, age-appropriate prompt that challenges the student to demonstrate the content and skill learned. Backup materials, self-checks, and rubrics are distributed along with the prompt and directions. Students plan their presentation with their peers, then present. This summative assessment is scored with a rubric and provides an end-of-unit grade (Connolly, 2020).

Performance Assessments

The **performance task** is the foundation of the skills-based summative assessment (see figure 5.2). It is considered an authentic assessment because it provides students with the opportunity to demonstrate what they have learned in both content and skill by creating a project or giving a demonstration.

A performance task requires active student engagement (see figure 5.5). It helps students envision the learning goals and makes clear what they are expected to know and be able to do. It challenges students to demonstrate what was learned when faced with a real-world, engaging prompt (Brookhart, 2024).

Student performance is enhanced when the teacher provides frequent formative assessment of the progress and gives effective feedback based on the performance indicators and the requirements of the task. The presentation is scored with a rubric and results in a grade.

Students demonstrate content and skills in a variety of ways. For example, the teacher may encourage students to demonstrate content and skills through role-play, a video, a public service announcement, a story, a poem, music, or an artistic representation such as a comic strip. To ensure success for all students, use the criteria of universal design for learning (UDL; see Universal Design for Learning later in this chapter) when planning (CAST, 2018). Students benefit from using a variety of performance assessment strategies because they use their talent to demonstrate content and skills, not just their ability to read or answer questions on a test (Connolly, 2020).

The following prompt is an example of using Standard 1 to teach about stress management. After explaining skills and strategies to reduce stress and support health and well-being (e.g., breathing, exercise, healthy eating, yoga, relaxation techniques), the teacher distributes the performance task, a self-check, backup materials, and the rubric.

Prompt

Aiden is feeling stressed. His parents go to work early and come home late. He gets up early with his parents so they can drive him to school, where he attends an "early bird special club." He also stays after school and participates in school clubs and activities. He takes the late bus home.

On weekends, he plays soccer in the fall, hockey in the winter, and baseball in the spring. He does not spend much time with his friends because he is too busy and too tired.

Lately, he feels anxious, has trouble concentrating, and gets stomachaches (Connolly, 2020, pp. 421-422).

Your challenge is to help Aiden improve his personal health by demonstrating practices that support health and well-being.

Your project includes:

1. A graphic organizer that explains two ways to manage stress. (Learning Indicator 1.5.3: "Explain ways to prevent or reduce risks for illnesses and injuries such as ways to manage chronic health conditions.")
2. Demonstrate two stress-reduction strategies that may help Aiden support his health and well-being. (Learning Indicator 7.5.2: "Demonstrate practices and behaviors that support health and well-being of self and others.") (SHAPE America, 2025).

FIGURE 5.5 Example of a performance task.

Rubrics

A **rubric** is a guide to score assessments. There are many types of rubrics, including but not limited to checklists; rating scales; structured observation guides; and descriptive, analytical, holistic, and single-point styles. The teacher designs a rubric that is consistent with the unit objectives and time available.

The criteria of the rubric consist of the content and skill performance indicators. Non-standard criteria such as neatness, voice projection, spelling, grammar, and so on are scored separately.

When designing a rubric, provide space to show the grade for each criterion, make comments, and provide feedback. This information is shared with the student and family and provides a foundation for conversation and improvement.

Rubrics are distributed with the performance task or earlier and provide clear performance expectations. Consequently, the student knows what is expected and what to do when demonstrating the content and skill.

Figure 5.6 is an example of an analytical rubric for the performance task example shown in figure 5.5.

Assessment Accommodations

Assessment accommodations are important when providing equal access to assessment for all students, particularly students with special needs or students with disabilities. The accommodations are informed by a student's individual

Score and feedback	Criteria	4	3	2	1	0
	1.5.3 Explain ways to prevent or reduce risks for illnesses and injuries *such as ways to manage chronic health conditions.*	The explanation of two ways to manage health conditions is accurate.	The explanation of two ways to manage health conditions is mostly accurate.	The explanation of two ways to manage health conditions has some inaccuracies.	The explanation of two ways to manage health conditions is inaccurate.	Not enough evidence to score.
	7.5.2 Demonstrate practices and behaviors that support health and well-being of self and others.	The demonstration of two stress-reduction strategies that support Aiden's health and well-being is accurate.	The demonstration of two stress-reduction strategies that support Aiden's health and well-being is mostly accurate.	The demonstration of two stress-reduction strategies that support Aiden's health and well-being has some inaccuracies.	The demonstration of two stress-reduction strategies that support Aiden's health and well-being is inaccurate.	Not enough evidence to score.
Total possible points – 8			Student score: ___/8 = Final grade			

FIGURE 5.6 A sample analytical rubric for the example performance task.

Note: Teachers may simplify the rubric language for students. However, the criteria and expectations must be consistent with the requirements of the performance task and indicators.

education plan (IEP) and 504 plan. Accommodations involve adjustments to the conditions or materials used in the assessment. Modifications include changes in the conditions or materials of the performance task (Brookhart, 2024).

An English language learner (ELL) also benefits from performance assessment and accommodations. The ELL may perform the Heimlich maneuver perfectly because of visually watching the skill and practicing. However, accommodations may be needed to complete a graphic organizer because of limited language skills.

Universal Design for Learning

When designing assessments, UDL provides accessibility with minimum accommodations. UDL removes barriers for all learners, regardless of the special need, language, or other issues.

UDL is intended to provide

- multiple means of engagement (the "why" of learning),
- multiple means of representation (the "what" of learning), and
- multiple means of action and expression (the "how" of learning) (CAST, 2018).

What do these criteria look like in a performance assessment?

- *Multiple means of engagement* (the "why" of learning) occurs when the teacher considers the students' interests, culture, personal relevance, subjectivity, effort, and background experiences as part of planning and assessment. The teacher helps the students stay focused and avoid distractions, clarifies the performance indicator objectives, encourages students to self-regulate, and provides effective feedback to enhance assessment performance.
- *Multiple means of representation* (the "what" of learning) occurs when the teacher uses a variety of strategies, including media, to teach students with auditory, visual, and learning disabilities, as well as those with language and cultural differences. Another strategy is to post key terms with corresponding pictures to facilitate understanding and learning.
- *Multiple means of action and expression* (the "how" of learning) occurs when the teacher provides different ways for the students to demonstrate content and skill performance indicators. Options include physical, verbal, and graphic expression using a variety of media and assistive technology (Brookhart, 2024).

Importance of Assessment

Assessments are used by students, teachers, districts, states, and national organizations for a variety of reasons.

Students use formative and summative assessments to determine what they need to know, how to improve, and what they need to do to reach the learning objectives of the units.

Assessment informs teachers of the individual needs of their students, identifies gaps in teaching and learning, and provides valuable information that determines if adjustments to teaching are needed.

Schools and districts use assessments to evaluate programs, examine teacher performance, and determine program resource needs and how best to support instruction.

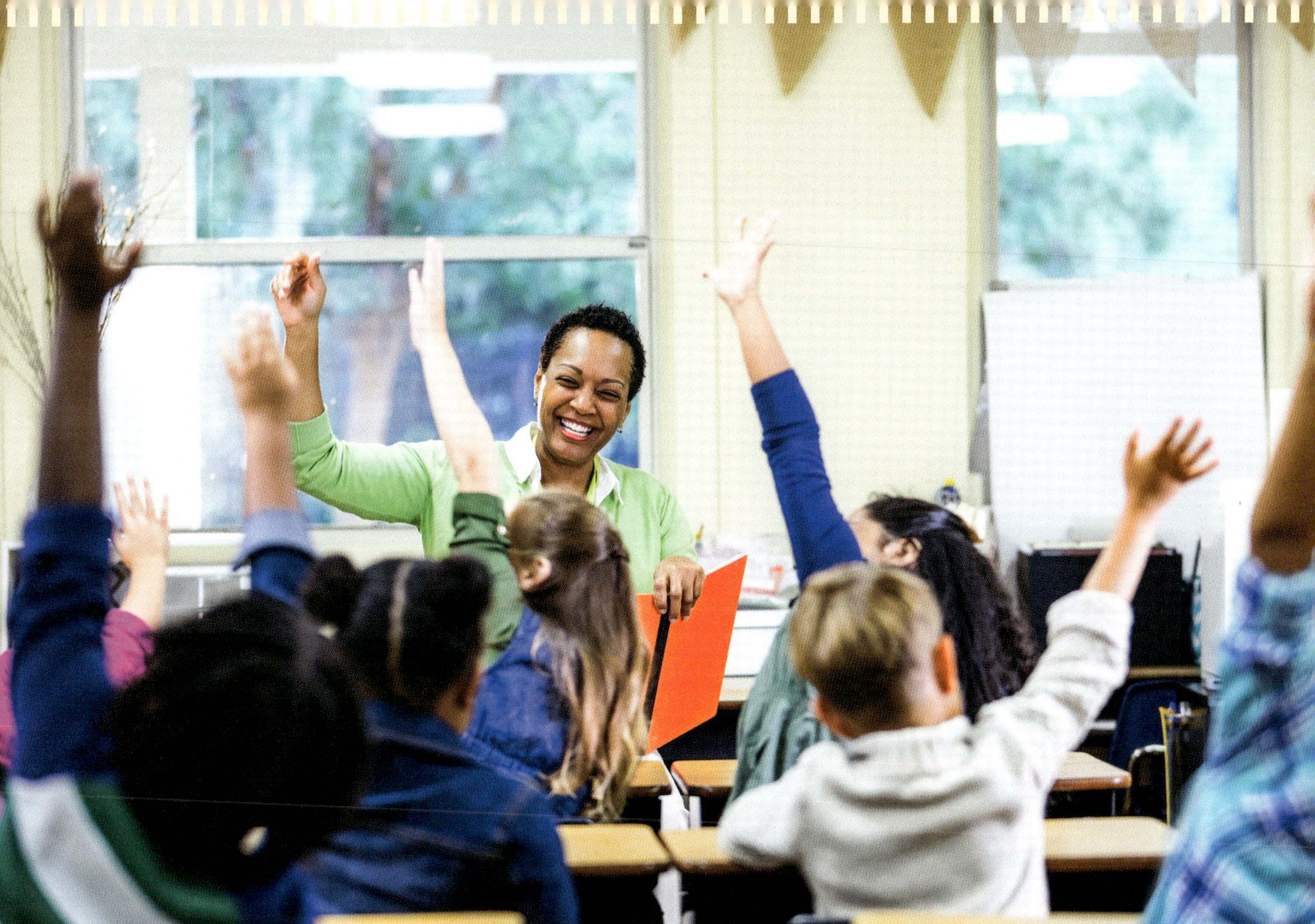

In states where health education is tested, assessment provides valuable information about student mastery of state standards that can be used to evaluate programs and initiatives (Institute of Educational Sciences, 2023).

Assessment is a vital component of a skills-based program. Examine a variety of in-seat and electronic formative assessments, and select those that help the students meet the learning goals. Plan authentic summative assessment based on the content and skills performance indicators. Provide time for students to plan and present. The data gained from the summative assessment help the teacher reflect on the efficacy of selected teaching strategies and gather student grades.

CHAPTER 6

A Closer Look at the Standards

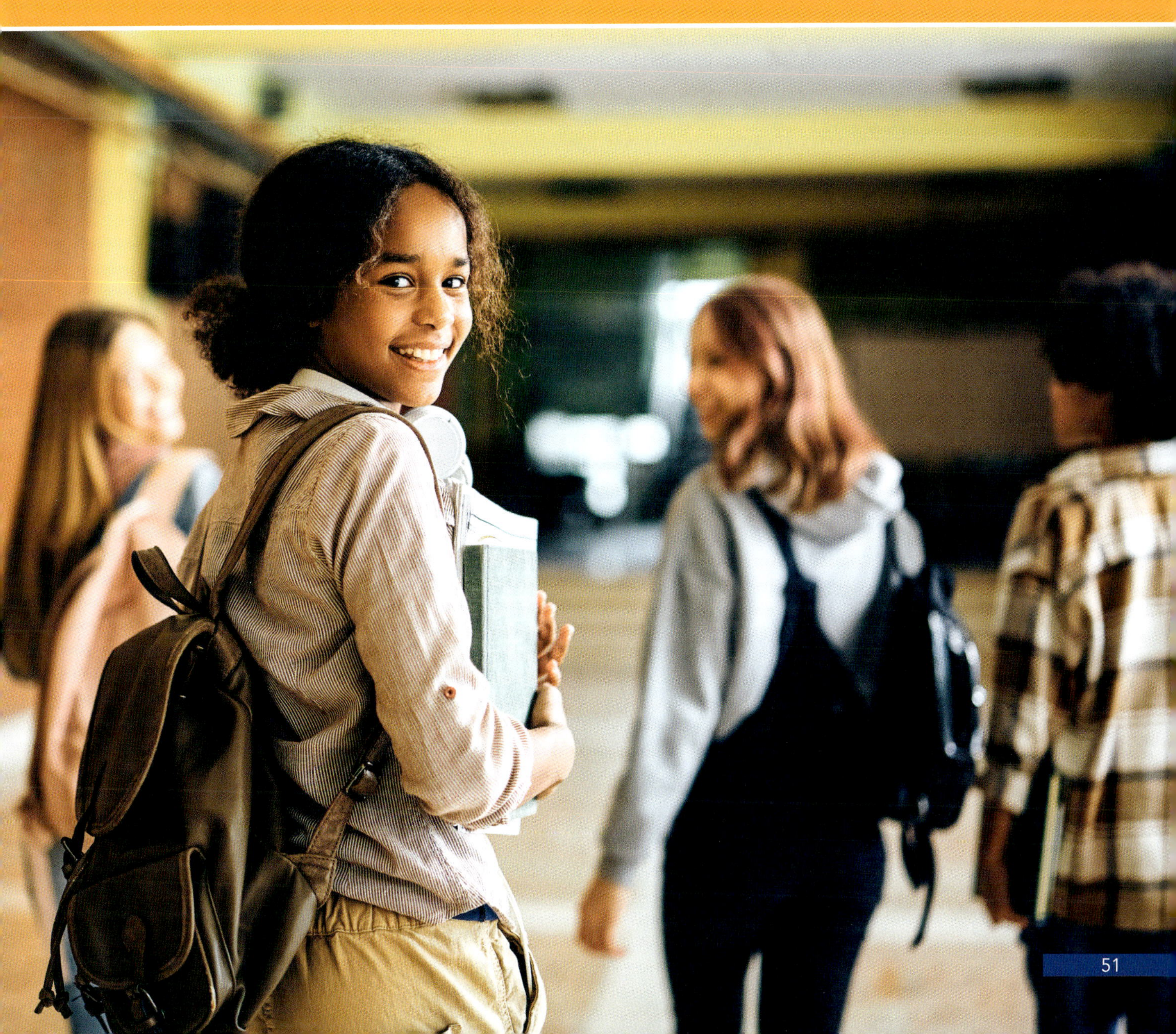

The 2024 SHAPE America National Health Education Standards document displays each standard (and its supporting information) as follows:

1. The standard
2. A rationale statement
3. Performance indicators (organized by grade span)

The Standards

Functional health information and underlying principles of health and well-being are included in Standard 1. Standards 2 to 8 identify skills that are applicable to overall health and well-being. These include identifying the impact of various influences on health behaviors; knowing how to access **valid** and **reliable** health resources; using interpersonal communication, decision-making, goal-setting, and advocacy skills; and practices to support the health of self and others.

Rationale Statements

A rationale statement is provided for each standard. The rationale illustrates the importance of each standard and is intended to provide additional clarity, direction, and understanding for how to teach and use the standard.

Performance Indicators

Performance indicators are provided for each of the National Health Education Standards, delineated by the following grade spans: grades preK to 2, grades 3 to 5, grades 6 to 8, and grades 9 to 12. Each performance indicator is introduced by this stem: "As a result of health instruction in [*grade span*], students will be able to . . ." The performance indicators are meant to be achieved by the end of the grade span in which they are identified.

Because learning best occurs when students perform at all levels of the cognitive domain, the performance indicators encompass application, analysis, synthesis, and evaluation, as well as knowledge and comprehension. Even primary grade students can learn at the higher levels of the cognitive domain if the concepts and learning activities are developmentally appropriate.

Performance indicators are also intended to serve as a blueprint for organizing student assessment. Student achievement of all performance indicators specified for each standard supports the successful attainment of that standard, ultimately increasing the likelihood that students will adopt and maintain healthy behaviors.

The standards, rationales, and performance indicators are first presented in order (Standards 1 to 8; see tables). For ease of identification, the performance indicators are numbered sequentially. Then, the standards and performance indicators are presented by each of the four grade spans (see "National Health Education Standards by Grade Span").

"Let us put our minds together and see what life we will make for our children."

Sitting Bull, chief of the Hunkpapa Lakota Nation

INDICATORS AT A GLANCE

Note: *This chart is intended to list the Grade-Span Performance Indicators for grades preK-12. This chart is not intended to show alignment across Grade-Span Performance Indicators. However, some indicators may align across grade spans and some may not due to the content and skills being taught within a specific grade span.*

STANDARD 1	Use functional health information to support health and well-being of self and others.		
RATIONALE	The acquisition and application of functional health information provides a foundation for promoting health and well-being. This standard includes essential concepts based on established theories and models of health behavior and **health promotion**. It focuses not only on risk factors, but also on protective factors that can support health and wellness. Concepts reflected in this standard include health literacy, health promotion, health equity, social determinants of health, well-being, and health outcomes within individual, interpersonal, community, societal, and environmental contexts. Functional information can be applied to health-related skills, such as analyzing influences, accessing resources, interpersonal communication, decision-making, goal-setting, engaging in health practices and behaviors, and advocacy.		
Grades preK-2 Performance Indicators	**Grades 3-5 Performance Indicators**	**Grades 6-8 Performance Indicators**	**Grades 9-12 Performance Indicators**
1.2.1 Identify strengths and assets that support health and well-being.	1.5.1 Explain how to build upon strengths and assets to support health and well-being.	1.8.1 Analyze ways to build upon strengths and assets to support individual and collective health and well-being.	1.12.1 Apply ways to build upon strengths and assets to support individual and collective health and well-being.
1.2.2 Identify dimensions of wellness.	1.5.2 Describe health-promoting behaviors for the dimensions of wellness.	1.8.2 Analyze how practices and behaviors support a variety of dimensions of wellness.	1.12.2 Analyze the relationships between various dimensions of wellness as related to health outcomes.
1.2.3 Identify ways to prevent or reduce risks for illnesses and injuries.	1.5.3 Explain ways to prevent or reduce risks for illnesses and injuries.	1.8.3 Analyze behaviors that reduce or prevent illnesses and injuries.	1.12.3 Evaluate behaviors that reduce or prevent illnesses and injuries.
1.2.4 Describe health-promoting behaviors.	1.5.4 Explain ways to engage in health-promoting behaviors, including how to manage health conditions.	1.8.4 Analyze practices and behaviors that support health and well-being, including how to manage health conditions.	1.12.4 Evaluate practices and behaviors that support health and well-being, including how to manage health conditions.
1.2.5 Explain the importance of health and well-being.	1.5.5 Examine how health literacy supports health and well-being.	1.8.5 Analyze connections between health literacy and health outcomes.	1.12.5 Examine connections between individual health literacy, organizational health literacy, and health outcomes.
1.2.6 Identify how the environment affects personal and community health.	1.5.6 Examine how the environment affects personal and community health.	1.8.6 Analyze how individual, interpersonal, community, and environmental factors impact health and well-being.	1.12.6 Analyze how individual, interpersonal, community, societal, and environmental factors are interrelated and impact health outcomes.

>continued

STANDARD 1 >*continued*

Grades preK-2 Performance Indicators	Grades 3-5 Performance Indicators	Grades 6-8 Performance Indicators	Grades 9-12 Performance Indicators
1.2.7 Explain when it is important to seek health care.	1.5.7 Explain when and why it is important to seek health care.	1.8.7 Explain how health care promotes personal health.	1.12.7 Analyze the benefits of and barriers to practicing a variety of health behaviors.
			1.12.8 Examine how self-efficacy, **perceived susceptibility, and perceived severity** affect health behaviors.
			1.12.9 Analyze the relationship between access to health care and overall health and well-being.

INDICATORS AT A GLANCE

Note: *This chart is intended to list the Grade-Span Performance Indicators for grades preK-12. This chart is not intended to show alignment across Grade-Span Performance Indicators. However, some indicators may align across grade spans and some may not due to the content and skills being taught within a specific grade span.*

STANDARD 2	Analyze influences that affect health and well-being of self and others.
RATIONALE	Health and well-being are affected by many, diverse influences within individual, interpersonal, community, societal, and environmental contexts. This standard focuses on identifying and evaluating internal and external factors influencing health practices and behaviors. Influences on health and well-being may include but are not limited to: personal values and beliefs, perceived and social norms, family, peers, schools, communities, culture, media and technology, policies, and the environment. This standard recognizes that the factors affecting health behaviors and outcomes, such as social determinants of health, are complex and impact people and communities differently. It also supports the individual's ability to identify and use skills to recognize the types of influences, analyze the role of influences across a variety of wellness dimensions, and manage influences on health and well-being in digital and in-person settings. This skill contributes to a better understanding of the connections between individual health, community health, and health equity, which can strengthen use of other health skills, such as accessing information and advocacy.

Grades preK-2 Performance Indicators	Grades 3-5 Performance Indicators	Grades 6-8 Performance Indicators	Grades 9-12 Performance Indicators
2.2.1 Identify various influences that affect health and well-being.	2.5.1 Explain how various influences affect health and well-being.	2.8.1 Analyze the interrelationships between various influences on health and well-being.	2.12.1 Evaluate the interrelationships and impacts of various influences and health behaviors on health and well-being.
2.2.2 Determine the ways various influences affect personal health and well-being.	2.5.2 Determine the ways various influences affect the health and well-being of self and others.	2.8.2 Analyze individual, interpersonal, community, societal, and environmental factors that influence health behaviors, health outcomes, and health equity.	2.12.2 Evaluate how social determinants of health influence health behaviors, health outcomes, and health equity.

Grades preK-2 Performance Indicators	Grades 3-5 Performance Indicators	Grades 6-8 Performance Indicators	Grades 9-12 Performance Indicators
2.2.3 Explain how various influences affect the health and well-being of others.	2.5.3 Explain how influences affect the health and well-being of people and communities in different ways.	2.8.3 Analyze how various influences affect the health and well-being of people and communities in different ways.	2.12.3 Evaluate how individual, interpersonal, community, societal, and environmental influences and factors affect health equity.
	2.5.4 Use strategies and resources to manage influences that impact health and well-being.	2.8.4 Apply strategies and resources to manage influences that impact health and well-being.	2.12.4 Formulate strategies to manage influences that impact health and well-being.
			2.12.5 Use resources to manage influences that impact health and well-being.

INDICATORS AT A GLANCE

Note: *This chart is intended to list the Grade-Span Performance Indicators for grades preK-12. This chart is not intended to show alignment across Grade-Span Performance Indicators. However, some indicators may align across grade spans and some may not due to the content and skills being taught within a specific grade span.*

STANDARD 3	Access valid and reliable resources to support health and well-being of self and others.		
RATIONALE	Access to valid and reliable health information, products, services, and other resources is essential to promoting health and well-being, and preventing, detecting, managing, and treating health issues and conditions. Access to valid and reliable information, products, services, and other resources promotes health and well-being in individual, interpersonal, community, societal, and environmental contexts. This standard focuses on identifying, accessing, and evaluating valid and reliable resources, including managing **misinformation** and **disinformation**, within digital and in-person settings. Media and technology play a significant and increasing role in the way individuals learn about and connect with ourselves, others, and the world. This standard engages students in critical thinking around media messages and resources, including how they are accessed, evaluated, and used to support health and well-being.		
Grades preK-2 Performance Indicators	**Grades 3-5 Performance Indicators**	**Grades 6-8 Performance Indicators**	**Grades 9-12 Performance Indicators**
3.2.1 Identify characteristics of trusted adults and other individuals who support health and well-being.	3.5.1 Determine which trusted adults, other individuals, and other health resources are appropriate in various situations.	3.8.1 Describe situations that may require support from trusted adults, other individuals, and health professionals.	3.12.1 Analyze the accessibility of trusted adults, other individuals, health professionals, and other resources to promote health and well-being.
3.2.2 Demonstrate when and how to seek help from others at home, at school, or in the community.	3.5.2 Locate home, school, and community resources to support health and well-being.	3.8.2 Identify supports and barriers to accessing valid and reliable health information, products, services, and other resources.	3.12.2 Analyze supports and barriers to accessing valid and reliable health information, products, services, and other resources.

>continued

STANDARD 3 >*continued*

Grades preK-2 Performance Indicators	Grades 3-5 Performance Indicators	Grades 6-8 Performance Indicators	Grades 9-12 Performance Indicators
3.2.3 Locate school and community **health helpers**.	3.5.3 Determine the validity and reliability of health information, products, services, and other resources.	3.8.3 Access valid and reliable sources of health information, products, services, and other resources.	3.12.3 Evaluate the validity, reliability, and accessibility of health information, products, services, and other resources.
	3.5.4 Explain how misinformation and disinformation affect health and well-being.	3.8.4 Analyze the validity, reliability, and accessibility of health information, products, services, and other resources.	3.12.4 Use valid and reliable sources of health information, products, services, and other resources.
		3.8.5 Use strategies to manage misinformation and disinformation.	3.12.5 Apply strategies to manage misinformation and disinformation.

INDICATORS AT A GLANCE

Note: *This chart is intended to list the Grade-Span Performance Indicators for grades preK-12. This chart is not intended to show alignment across Grade-Span Performance Indicators. However, some indicators may align across grade spans and some may not due to the content and skills being taught within a specific grade span.*

STANDARD 4	Use interpersonal communication skills to support health and well-being of self and others.
RATIONALE	Effective communication promotes health and well-being in individual, interpersonal, community, societal, and environmental contexts. This standard focuses on expressive and receptive communication in digital and in-person settings. Combined with perspective-taking, communication skills help to recognize and strengthen interpersonal interactions, create and maintain relationships, express and interpret messages, and manage conflict. Developing communication skills helps individuals to see how they communicate and the ways in which their communication affects those around them.

Grades preK-2 Performance Indicators	Grades 3-5 Performance Indicators	Grades 6-8 Performance Indicators	Grades 9-12 Performance Indicators
4.2.1 Express thoughts, feelings, wants, and needs to support health and well-being of self and others.	4.5.1 Use effective communication skills to express thoughts, feelings, wants, and needs to support health and well-being of self and others.	4.8.1 Use effective communication skills across various modes of communication to support health and well-being of self and others.	4.12.1 Apply effective communication skills across multiple modes of communication and media formats to support health and well-being of self and others.
4.2.2 Use active listening skills in a variety of situations.	4.5.2 Use active listening skills and strategies in a variety of situations.	4.8.2 Apply active listening skills and strategies in a variety of interpersonal contexts.	4.12.2 Apply communication skills and strategies within a variety of interpersonal contexts.
4.2.3 Demonstrate communication skills and strategies to use if uncomfortable, unsafe, or harmed.	4.5.3 Demonstrate how to ask for and offer assistance to support the health of self and others.	4.8.3 Use various communication strategies to seek and offer support and assistance.	4.12.3 Demonstrate how to ask for and offer assistance to support the health of self and others.

Grades preK-2 Performance Indicators	Grades 3-5 Performance Indicators	Grades 6-8 Performance Indicators	Grades 9-12 Performance Indicators
4.2.4 Recognize ways to communicate and respect the boundaries of self and others.	4.5.4 Demonstrate boundary-setting skills to communicate and respect the boundaries of self and others.	4.8.4 Demonstrate ways to communicate boundaries and consent for a variety of situations.	4.12.4 Use communication skills related to communicating boundaries, expressing consent, and removing consent in a variety of situations.
4.2.5 Demonstrate ways to show kindness and compassion.	4.5.5 Demonstrate refusal skills to use in a variety of situations.	4.8.5 Use refusal skills and strategies in a variety of situations.	4.12.5 Apply refusal skills and strategies in a variety of situations.
	4.5.6 Demonstrate strategies to prevent, manage, or resolve conflict.	4.8.6 Use skills and strategies to prevent, manage, or resolve conflict.	4.12.6 Apply skills and strategies to prevent, manage, or resolve conflict.
	4.5.7 Demonstrate effective ways to communicate with kindness and compassion.	4.8.7 Use collaboration skills in a variety of situations.	4.12.7 Demonstrate collaboration skills in a variety of situations.
		4.8.8 Use negotiation skills in a variety of situations.	4.12.8 Demonstrate negotiation skills in a variety of situations.
		4.8.9 Demonstrate strategies to communicate with others with different perspectives and values.	4.12.9 Adapt strategies to communicate with others with different perspectives and values in various contexts.
		4.8.10 Demonstrate ways to communicate empathy and compassion.	4.12.10 Communicate with empathy and compassion.

INDICATORS AT A GLANCE

Note: *This chart is intended to list the Grade-Span Performance Indicators for grades preK-12. This chart is not intended to show alignment across Grade-Span Performance Indicators. However, some indicators may align across grade spans and some may not due to the content and skills being taught within a specific grade span.*

STANDARD 5	Use a decision-making process to support health and well-being of self and others.		
RATIONALE	Effective decision-making is needed to identify, adopt, and maintain health-promoting behaviors. This standard includes skills and steps integral to the process of effective decision-making to support health and well-being. The decision-making process enables collaboration to improve quality of life within individual, interpersonal, community, societal, and environmental contexts.		
Grades preK-2 Performance Indicators	**Grades 3-5 Performance Indicators**	**Grades 6-8 Performance Indicators**	**Grades 9-12 Performance Indicators**
5.2.1 Identify when a health-related decision is needed to maintain or improve health and well-being.	5.5.1 Determine situations that require a thoughtful decision-making process to maintain or improve health and well-being.	5.8.1 Explain how the use of a decision-making process affects health and well-being.	5.12.1 Analyze how health-related decisions may affect personal and community health and well-being from a variety of perspectives.

>continued

STANDARD 5 >*continued*

Grades preK-2 Performance Indicators	Grades 3-5 Performance Indicators	Grades 6-8 Performance Indicators	Grades 9-12 Performance Indicators
5.2.2 Recognize when help is needed for a health-related decision.	5.5.2 Determine whether assistance or collaboration is needed in making a health-related decision.	5.8.2 Determine when health-related situations require the application of a thoughtful decision-making process.	5.12.2 Determine when and why health-related situations require the application of a thoughtful decision-making process.
5.2.3 Describe options and potential outcomes for a health-related decision.	5.5.3 Compare and contrast options and potential outcomes for a health-related decision.	5.8.3 Use an individual, supported, or collaborative decision-making process to maintain or improve health and well-being.	5.12.3 Apply an individual, supported, or collaborative decision-making process to maintain or improve health and well-being.
5.2.4 Choose an option that supports health and well-being.	5.5.4 Choose a health-promoting option when making a decision.	5.8.4 Evaluate how various options may affect health-related outcomes at individual, interpersonal, community, societal, and environmental levels.	5.12.4 Analyze a variety of options based on priorities and potential outcomes when making a health-related decision.
	5.5.5 Reflect on the results of a health-related decision on self and others.	5.8.5 Identify supports and barriers that affect decision making at individual, interpersonal, community, societal, and environmental levels.	5.12.5 Analyze the potential impact of a decision on the health and well-being at individual, interpersonal, community, societal, and environmental levels.
		5.8.6 Evaluate the results of a health-related decision on self and others.	5.12.6 Develop a plan of action to implement a health-related decision.
			5.12.7 Evaluate the impact of supports and barriers that affect decision making at individual, interpersonal, community, societal, and environmental levels.
			5.12.8 Evaluate the effectiveness of health-related decisions.

INDICATORS AT A GLANCE

Note: *This chart is intended to list the Grade-Span Performance Indicators for grades preK-12. This chart is not intended to show alignment across Grade-Span Performance Indicators. However, some indicators may align across grade spans and some may not due to the content and skills being taught within a specific grade span.*

STANDARD 6	Use a goal-setting process to support health and well-being of self and others.		
RATIONALE	Goal-setting is a process to support short- and long-term health and well-being goals. In addition to achieving a goal, a goal-setting process includes using practices, habits, and routines in daily life. This standard includes the processes needed to plan, reach, and reflect on health goals. Setting goals is a flexible process, and considers personal and social factors affecting health and well-being. Goal-setting supports aspirations and future planning for health and well-being within individual, interpersonal, community, societal, and environmental contexts.		
Grades preK-2 Performance Indicators	**Grades 3-5 Performance Indicators**	**Grades 6-8 Performance Indicators**	**Grades 9-12 Performance Indicators**
6.2.1 Determine a health behavior to change or reinforce.	6.5.1 Set a goal and explain how the goal supports health and well-being.	6.8.1 Assess personal health and well-being to identify focus areas for goal-setting.	6.12.1 Assess personal health, well-being, and factors for engaging in a goal-setting process.
6.2.2 Identify a goal that supports health and well-being.	6.5.2 Determine whether assistance or collaboration is needed in setting a goal that supports health and well-being.	6.8.2 Analyze when individual, supported, or collaborative goal-setting is appropriate.	6.12.2 Use an individual, supported, or collaborative goal-setting process as appropriate.
6.2.3 Determine who can help when assistance is needed to achieve a health-related goal.	6.5.3 Develop a plan that includes actions, resources, and progress-tracking toward attaining a health-related goal.	6.8.3 Develop a goal and explain how it supports health and well-being.	6.12.3 Develop a goal and analyze how it supports health and well-being.
6.2.4 Describe actions that support reaching a health-related goal.	6.5.4 Identify supports and barriers that affect progress toward attaining a health-related goal.	6.8.4 Develop a plan that addresses supports and barriers to attaining a health-related goal.	6.12.4 Implement a plan that addresses supports and barriers to attaining a health-related goal.
6.2.5 Take action to achieve a health-related goal.	6.5.5 Track progress toward attaining a health-related goal.	6.8.5 Monitor progress to determine whether a health-related goal or plan should be maintained or adjusted.	6.12.5 Monitor progress and adjust the goal or plan as appropriate.
6.2.6 Reflect on the results of goal-setting.	6.5.6 Reflect on the goal-setting process and outcomes.	6.8.6 Examine the goal-setting process and outcomes on health and well-being.	6.12.6 Evaluate the goal-setting process and outcomes on health and well-being.

INDICATORS AT A GLANCE

Note: *This chart is intended to list the Grade-Span Performance Indicators for grades preK-12. This chart is not intended to show alignment across Grade-Span Performance Indicators. However, some indicators may align across grade spans and some may not due to the content and skills being taught within a specific grade span.*

STANDARD 7	Demonstrate practices and behaviors to support health and well-being of self and others.		
RATIONALE	Developing health practices and behaviors can promote health and well-being over the lifespan and reduce risk to self and others. Practicing health behaviors is critical to incorporating health-promoting habits and routines into all dimensions of wellness. Due to the increasing influence of technology, it is crucial to develop and apply practices and behaviors that support media balance and digital wellness. This standard promotes individual and collective responsibility by encouraging the exploration and practice of skills and processes that support health and well-being in individual, interpersonal, community, societal, and environmental contexts.		
Grades preK-2 Performance Indicators	**Grades 3-5 Performance Indicators**	**Grades 6-8 Performance Indicators**	**Grades 9-12 Performance Indicators**
7.2.1 Identify practices and behaviors that support health and well-being of self and others.	7.5.1 Examine practices and behaviors that support health and well-being of self and others.	7.8.1 Examine supports and barriers to health-related practices and behaviors.	7.12.1 Analyze supports and barriers to engaging in health-related practices and behaviors.
7.2.2 Demonstrate practices and behaviors that support health and well-being of self and others.	7.5.2 Demonstrate practices and behaviors that support health and well-being of self and others.	7.8.2 Analyze practices and behaviors that support personal and community health and well-being.	7.12.2 Evaluate practices, behaviors, and other factors supporting individual and collective health and well-being.
		7.8.3 Demonstrate practices and behaviors that support personal and community health and well-being.	7.12.3 Adapt practices and behaviors to support individual and collective health and well-being.
			7.12.4 Demonstrate a variety of practices and behaviors supporting individual and collective health and well-being.

INDICATORS AT A GLANCE

Note: *This chart is intended to list the Grade-Span Performance Indicators for grades preK-12. This chart is not intended to show alignment across Grade-Span Performance Indicators. However, some indicators may align across grade spans and some may not due to the content and skills being taught within a specific grade span.*

STANDARD 8	Advocate to promote health and well-being of self and others.		
RATIONALE	Advocacy skills are critical for promoting health and well-being within individual, interpersonal, community, societal, and environmental contexts. This standard helps learners develop and apply skills and strategies to increase agency and advocacy for self and others. Practicing advocacy helps students be informed, civic-minded members of their community, who are inclusive of individual, cultural, historical, and other differences.		
Grades preK-2 Performance Indicators	**Grades 3-5 Performance Indicators**	**Grades 6-8 Performance Indicators**	**Grades 9-12 Performance Indicators**
8.2.1 Make requests to support personal health and well-being.	8.5.1 Recognize situations in which advocacy supports the health and well-being of self and others.	8.8.1 Analyze opportunities to advocate for the health and well-being of individuals, families, and communities.	8.12.1 Examine a variety of factors that affect advocacy at individual, interpersonal, community, societal, and environmental levels.
8.2.2 Identify a variety of ways to support others in making health-promoting choices.	8.5.2 Explain how collaboration and communication support advocacy.	8.8.2 Determine when individual or collaborative advocacy is appropriate to promote health and well-being.	8.12.2 Advocate for health issues either collaboratively or individually to promote health and well-being.
8.2.3 Encourage others to make health-promoting choices.	8.5.3 Identify advocacy skills and strategies to support health and well-being.	8.8.3 Adapt advocacy skills and strategies for a variety of audiences and contexts.	8.12.3 Customize advocacy skills and strategies for varying audiences and contexts.
	8.5.4 Demonstrate how to advocate for health and well-being.	8.8.4 Demonstrate advocacy skills and strategies to promote the health and well-being of self and others.	8.12.4 Demonstrate self-advocacy skills and strategies to promote health and well-being.
		8.8.5 Evaluate the effectiveness of advocacy efforts for promoting health and well-being.	8.12.5 Demonstrate advocacy skills and strategies to promote health and well-being at interpersonal, community, societal, and environmental levels.
			8.12.6 Evaluate the process, outcomes, and impact of advocacy efforts at the individual, interpersonal, community, societal, and environmental levels.
			8.12.7 Analyze the role of collaboration among different people in a community to prevent and solve community health issues.

National Health Education Standards by Grade Span

INDICATORS AT A GLANCE

Note: *This chart is intended to list the Standard Performance Indicators for grades preK-2. This chart is not intended to show alignment across Standard Performance Indicators. However, some indicators may align across standards and some may not due to the content and skills being taught within a specific standard.*

GRADES PREK-2	
STANDARD 1	Use functional health information to support health and well-being of self and others.
1.2.1	Identify strengths and assets that support health and well-being.
1.2.2	Identify dimensions of wellness.
1.2.3	Identify ways to prevent or reduce risks for illnesses and injuries.
1.2.4	Describe health-promoting behaviors.
1.2.5	Explain the importance of health and well-being.
1.2.6	Identify how the environment affects personal and community health.
1.2.7	Explain when it is important to seek health care.
STANDARD 2	Analyze influences that affect health and well-being of self and others.
2.2.1	Identify various influences that affect health and well-being.
2.2.2	Determine the ways various influences affect personal health and well-being.
2.2.3	Explain how various influences affect the health and well-being of others.
STANDARD 3	Access valid and reliable resources to support health and well-being of self and others.
3.2.1	Identify characteristics of trusted adults and other individuals who support health and well-being.
3.2.2	Demonstrate when and how to seek help from others at home, at school, or in the community.
3.2.3	Locate school and community health helpers.
STANDARD 4	Use interpersonal communication skills to support health and well-being of self and others.
4.2.1	Express thoughts, feelings, wants, and needs to support health and well-being of self and others.
4.2.2	Use active listening skills in a variety of situations.
4.2.3	Demonstrate communication skills and strategies to use if uncomfortable, unsafe, or harmed.
4.2.4	Recognize ways to communicate and respect the boundaries of self and others.
4.2.5	Demonstrate ways to show kindness and compassion.
STANDARD 5	Use a decision-making process to support health and well-being of self and others.
5.2.1	Identify when a health-related decision is needed to maintain or improve health and well-being.
5.2.2	Recognize when help is needed for a health-related decision.
5.2.3	Describe options and potential outcomes for a health-related decision.
5.2.4	Choose an option that supports health and well-being.
STANDARD 6	Use a goal-setting process to support health and well-being of self and others.
6.2.1	Determine a health behavior to change or reinforce.
6.2.2	Identify a goal that supports health and well-being.
6.2.3	Determine who can help when assistance is needed to achieve a health-related goal.
6.2.4	Describe actions that support reaching a health-related goal.
6.2.5	Take action to achieve a health-related goal.
6.2.6	Reflect on the results of goal-setting.

STANDARD 7	Demonstrate practices and behaviors to support health and well-being of self and others.
7.2.1	Identify practices and behaviors that support health and well-being of self and others.
7.2.2	Demonstrate practices and behaviors that support health and well-being of self and others.
STANDARD 8	Advocate to promote health and well-being of self and others.
8.2.1	Make requests to support personal health and well-being.
8.2.2	Identify a variety of ways to support others in making health-promoting choices.
8.2.3	Encourage others to make health-promoting choices.

INDICATORS AT A GLANCE

Note: *This chart is intended to list the Standard Performance Indicators for grades 3-5. This chart is not intended to show alignment across Standard Performance Indicators. However, some indicators may align across standards and some may not due to the content and skills being taught within a specific standard.*

GRADES 3-5	
STANDARD 1	Use functional health information to support health and well-being of self and others.
1.5.1	Explain how to build upon strengths and assets to support health and well-being.
1.5.2	Describe health-promoting behaviors for the dimensions of wellness.
1.5.3	Explain ways to prevent or reduce risks for illnesses and injuries.
1.5.4	Explain ways to engage in health-promoting behaviors, including how to manage health conditions.
1.5.5	Examine how health literacy supports health and well-being.
1.5.6	Examine how the environment affects personal and community health.
1.5.7	Explain when and why it is important to seek health care.
STANDARD 2	Analyze influences that affect health and well-being of self and others.
2.5.1	Explain how various influences affect health and well-being.
2.5.2	Determine the ways various influences affect the health and well-being of self and others.
2.5.3	Explain how influences affect the health and well-being of people and communities in different ways.
2.5.4	Use strategies and resources to manage influences that impact health and well-being.
STANDARD 3	Access valid and reliable resources to support health and well-being of self and others.
3.5.1	Determine which trusted adults, other individuals, and other health resources are appropriate in various situations.
3.5.2	Locate home, school, and community resources to support health and well-being.
3.5.3	Determine the validity and reliability of health information, products, services, and other resources.
3.5.4	Explain how misinformation and disinformation affect health and well-being.
STANDARD 4	Use interpersonal communication skills to support health and well-being of self and others.
4.5.1	Use effective communication skills to express thoughts, feelings, wants, and needs to support health and well-being of self and others.
4.5.2	Use active listening skills and strategies in a variety of situations.
4.5.3	Demonstrate how to ask for and offer assistance to support the health of self and others.
4.5.4	Demonstrate boundary-setting skills to communicate and respect the boundaries of self and others.
4.5.5	Demonstrate refusal skills to use in a variety of situations.
4.5.6	Demonstrate strategies to prevent, manage, or resolve conflict.
4.5.7	Demonstrate effective ways to communicate with kindness and compassion.

>*continued*

GRADES 3-5 >*continued*

STANDARD 5	Use a decision-making process to support health and well-being of self and others.
5.5.1	Determine situations that require a thoughtful decision-making process to maintain or improve health and well-being.
5.5.2	Determine whether assistance or collaboration is needed in making a health-related decision.
5.5.3	Compare and contrast options and potential outcomes for a health-related decision.
5.5.4	Choose a health-promoting option when making a decision.
5.5.5	Reflect on the results of a health-related decision on self and others.
STANDARD 6	Use a goal-setting process to support health and well-being of self and others.
6.5.1	Set a goal and explain how the goal supports health and well-being.
6.5.2	Determine whether assistance or collaboration is needed in setting a goal that supports health and well-being.
6.5.3	Develop a plan that includes actions, resources, and progress-tracking toward attaining a health-related goal.
6.5.4	Identify supports and barriers that affect progress toward attaining a health-related goal.
6.5.5	Track progress toward attaining a health-related goal.
6.5.6	Reflect on the goal-setting process and outcomes.
STANDARD 7	Demonstrate practices and behaviors to support health and well-being of self and others.
7.5.1	Examine practices and behaviors that support health and well-being of self and others.
7.5.2	Demonstrate practices and behaviors that support health and well-being of self and others.
STANDARD 8	Advocate to promote health and well-being of self and others.
8.5.1	Recognize situations in which advocacy supports the health and well-being of self and others.
8.5.2	Explain how collaboration and communication support advocacy.
8.5.3	Identify advocacy skills and strategies to support health and well-being.
8.5.4	Demonstrate how to advocate for health and well-being.

INDICATORS AT A GLANCE

Note: *This chart is intended to list the Standard Performance Indicators for grades 6-8. This chart is not intended to show alignment across Standard Performance Indicators. However, some indicators may align across standards and some may not due to the content and skills being taught within a specific standard.*

GRADES 6-8	
STANDARD 1	Use functional health information to support health and well-being of self and others.
1.8.1	Analyze ways to build upon strengths and assets to support individual and collective health and well-being.
1.8.2	Analyze how practices and behaviors support a variety of dimensions of wellness.
1.8.3	Analyze behaviors that reduce or prevent illnesses and injuries.
1.8.4	Analyze practices and behaviors that support health and well-being, including how to manage health conditions.
1.8.5	Analyze connections between health literacy and health outcomes.
1.8.6	Analyze how individual, interpersonal, community, and environmental factors impact health and well-being.
1.8.7	Explain how health care promotes personal health.

STANDARD 2	Analyze influences that affect health and well-being of self and others.
2.8.1	Analyze the interrelationships between various influences on health and well-being.
2.8.2	Analyze individual, interpersonal, community, societal, and environmental factors that influence health behaviors, health outcomes, and health equity.
2.8.3	Analyze how various influences affect the health and well-being of people and communities in different ways.
2.8.4	Apply strategies and resources to manage influences that impact health and well-being.
STANDARD 3	Access valid and reliable resources to support health and well-being of self and others.
3.8.1	Describe situations that may require support from trusted adults, other individuals, and health professionals.
3.8.2	Identify supports and barriers to accessing valid and reliable health information, products, services, and other resources.
3.8.3	Access valid and reliable sources of health information, products, services, and other resources.
3.8.4	Analyze the validity, reliability, and accessibility of health information, products, services, and other resources.
3.8.5	Use strategies to manage misinformation and disinformation.
STANDARD 4	Use interpersonal communication skills to support health and well-being of self and others.
4.8.1	Use effective communication skills across various modes of communication to support health and well-being of self and others.
4.8.2	Apply active listening skills and strategies in a variety of interpersonal contexts.
4.8.3	Use various communication strategies to seek and offer support and assistance.
4.8.4	Demonstrate ways to communicate boundaries and consent for a variety of situations.
4.8.5	Use refusal skills and strategies in a variety of situations.
4.8.6	Use skills and strategies to prevent, manage, or resolve conflict.
4.8.7	Use collaboration skills in a variety of situations.
4.8.8	Use negotiation skills in a variety of situations.
4.8.9	Demonstrate strategies to communicate with others with different perspectives and values.
4.8.10	Demonstrate ways to communicate empathy and compassion.
STANDARD 5	Use a decision-making process to support health and well-being of self and others.
5.8.1	Explain how the use of a decision-making process affects health and well-being.
5.8.2	Determine when health-related situations require the application of a thoughtful decision-making process.
5.8.3	Use an individual, supported, or collaborative decision-making process to maintain or improve health and well-being.
5.8.4	Evaluate how various options may affect health-related outcomes at individual, interpersonal, community, societal, and environmental levels.
5.8.5	Identify supports and barriers that affect decision making at individual, interpersonal, community, societal, and environmental levels.
5.8.6	Evaluate the results of a health-related decision on self and others.

>continued

GRADES 6-8 *>continued*

STANDARD 6	Use a goal-setting process to support health and well-being of self and others.
6.8.1	Assess personal health and well-being to identify focus areas for goal-setting.
6.8.2	Analyze when individual, supported, or collaborative goal-setting is appropriate.
6.8.3	Develop a goal and explain how it supports health and well-being.
6.8.4	Develop a plan that addresses supports and barriers to attaining a health-related goal.
6.8.5	Monitor progress to determine whether a health-related goal or plan should be maintained or adjusted.
6.8.6	Examine the goal-setting process and outcomes on health and well-being.
STANDARD 7	Demonstrate practices and behaviors to support health and well-being of self and others.
7.8.1	Examine supports and barriers to health-related practices and behaviors.
7.8.2	Analyze practices and behaviors that support personal and community health and well-being.
7.8.3	Demonstrate practices and behaviors that support personal and community health and well-being.
STANDARD 8	Advocate to promote health and well-being of self and others.
8.8.1	Analyze opportunities to advocate for the health and well-being of individuals, families, and communities.
8.8.2	Determine when individual or collaborative advocacy is appropriate to promote health and well-being.
8.8.3	Adapt advocacy skills and strategies for a variety of audiences and contexts.
8.8.4	Demonstrate advocacy skills and strategies to promote the health and well-being of self and others.
8.8.5	Evaluate the effectiveness of advocacy efforts for promoting health and well-being.

INDICATORS AT A GLANCE

Note: *This chart is intended to list the Standard Performance Indicators for grades 9-12. This chart is not intended to show alignment across Standard Performance Indicators. However, some indicators may align across standards and some may not due to the content and skills being taught within a specific standard.*

GRADES 9-12	
STANDARD 1	Use functional health information to support health and well-being of self and others.
1.12.1	Apply ways to build upon strengths and assets to support individual and collective health and well-being.
1.12.2	Analyze the relationships between various dimensions of wellness as related to health outcomes.
1.12.3	Evaluate behaviors that reduce or prevent illnesses and injuries.
1.12.4	Evaluate practices and behaviors that support health and well-being, including how to manage health conditions.
1.12.5	Examine connections between individual health literacy, organizational health literacy, and health outcomes.
1.12.6	Analyze how individual, interpersonal, community, societal, and environmental factors are interrelated and impact health outcomes.
1.12.7	Analyze the benefits of and barriers to practicing a variety of health behaviors.
1.12.8	Examine how self-efficacy, perceived susceptibility, and perceived severity affect health behaviors.
1.12.9	Analyze the relationship between access to health care and overall health and well-being.

STANDARD 2	Analyze influences that affect health and well-being of self and others.
2.12.1	Evaluate the interrelationships and impacts of various influences and health behaviors on health and well-being.
2.12.2	Evaluate how social determinants of health influence health behaviors, health outcomes, and health equity.
2.12.3	Evaluate how individual, interpersonal, community, societal, and environmental influences and factors affect health equity.
2.12.4	Formulate strategies to manage influences that impact health and well-being.
2.12.5	Use resources to manage influences that impact health and well-being.
STANDARD 3	Access valid and reliable resources to support health and well-being of self and others.
3.12.1	Analyze the accessibility of trusted adults, other individuals, health professionals, and other resources to promote health and well-being.
3.12.2	Analyze supports and barriers to accessing valid and reliable health information, products, services, and other resources.
3.12.3	Evaluate the validity, reliability, and accessibility of health information, products, services, and other resources.
3.12.4	Use valid and reliable sources of health information, products, services, and other resources.
3.12.5	Apply strategies to manage misinformation and disinformation.
STANDARD 4	Use interpersonal communication skills to support health and well-being of self and others.
4.12.1	Apply effective communication skills across multiple modes of communication and media formats to support health and well-being of self and others.
4.12.2	Apply communication skills and strategies within a variety of interpersonal contexts.
4.12.3	Demonstrate how to ask for and offer assistance to support the health of self and others.
4.12.4	Use communication skills related to communicating boundaries, expressing consent, and removing consent in a variety of situations.
4.12.5	Apply refusal skills and strategies in a variety of situations.
4.12.6	Apply skills and strategies to prevent, manage, or resolve conflict.
4.12.7	Demonstrate collaboration skills in a variety of situations.
4.12.8	Demonstrate negotiation skills in a variety of situations.
4.12.9	Adapt strategies to communicate with others with different perspectives and values in various contexts.
4.12.10	Communicate with empathy and compassion.
STANDARD 5	Use a decision-making process to support health and well-being of self and others.
5.12.1	Analyze how health-related decisions may affect personal and community health and well-being from a variety of perspectives.
5.12.2	Determine when and why health-related situations require the application of a thoughtful decision-making process.
5.12.3	Apply an individual, supported, or collaborative decision-making process to maintain or improve health and well-being.
5.12.4	Analyze a variety of options based on priorities and potential outcomes when making a health-related decision.
5.12.5	Analyze the potential impact of a decision on the health and well-being at individual, interpersonal, community, societal, and environmental levels.
5.12.6	Develop a plan of action to implement a health-related decision.
5.12.7	Evaluate the impact of supports and barriers that affect decision making at individual, interpersonal, community, societal, and environmental levels.
5.12.8	Evaluate the effectiveness of health-related decisions.

>continued

GRADES 9-12 >*continued*

STANDARD 6	Use a goal-setting process to support health and well-being of self and others.
6.12.1	Assess personal health, well-being, and factors for engaging in a goal-setting process.
6.12.2	Use an individual, supported, or collaborative goal-setting process as appropriate.
6.12.3	Develop a goal and analyze how it supports health and well-being.
6.12.4	Implement a plan that addresses supports and barriers to attaining a health-related goal.
6.12.5	Monitor progress and adjust the goal or plan as appropriate.
6.12.6	Evaluate the goal-setting process and outcomes on health and well-being.
STANDARD 7	Demonstrate practices and behaviors to support health and well-being of self and others.
7.12.1	Analyze supports and barriers to engaging in health-related practices and behaviors.
7.12.2	Evaluate practices, behaviors, and other factors supporting individual and collective health and well-being.
7.12.3	Adapt practices and behaviors to support individual and collective health and well-being.
7.12.4	Demonstrate a variety of practices and behaviors supporting individual and collective health and well-being.
STANDARD 8	Advocate to promote health and well-being of self and others.
8.12.1	Examine a variety of factors that affect advocacy at individual, interpersonal, community, societal, and environmental levels.
8.12.2	Advocate for health issues either collaboratively or individually to promote health and well-being.
8.12.3	Customize advocacy skills and strategies for varying audiences and contexts.
8.12.4	Demonstrate self-advocacy skills and strategies to promote health and well-being.
8.12.5	Demonstrate advocacy skills and strategies to promote health and well-being at interpersonal, community, societal, and environmental levels.
8.12.6	Evaluate the process, outcomes, and impact of advocacy efforts at the individual, interpersonal, community, societal, and environmental levels.
8.12.7	Analyze the role of collaboration among different people in a community to prevent and solve community health issues.

CHAPTER 7

Background on Standards Development

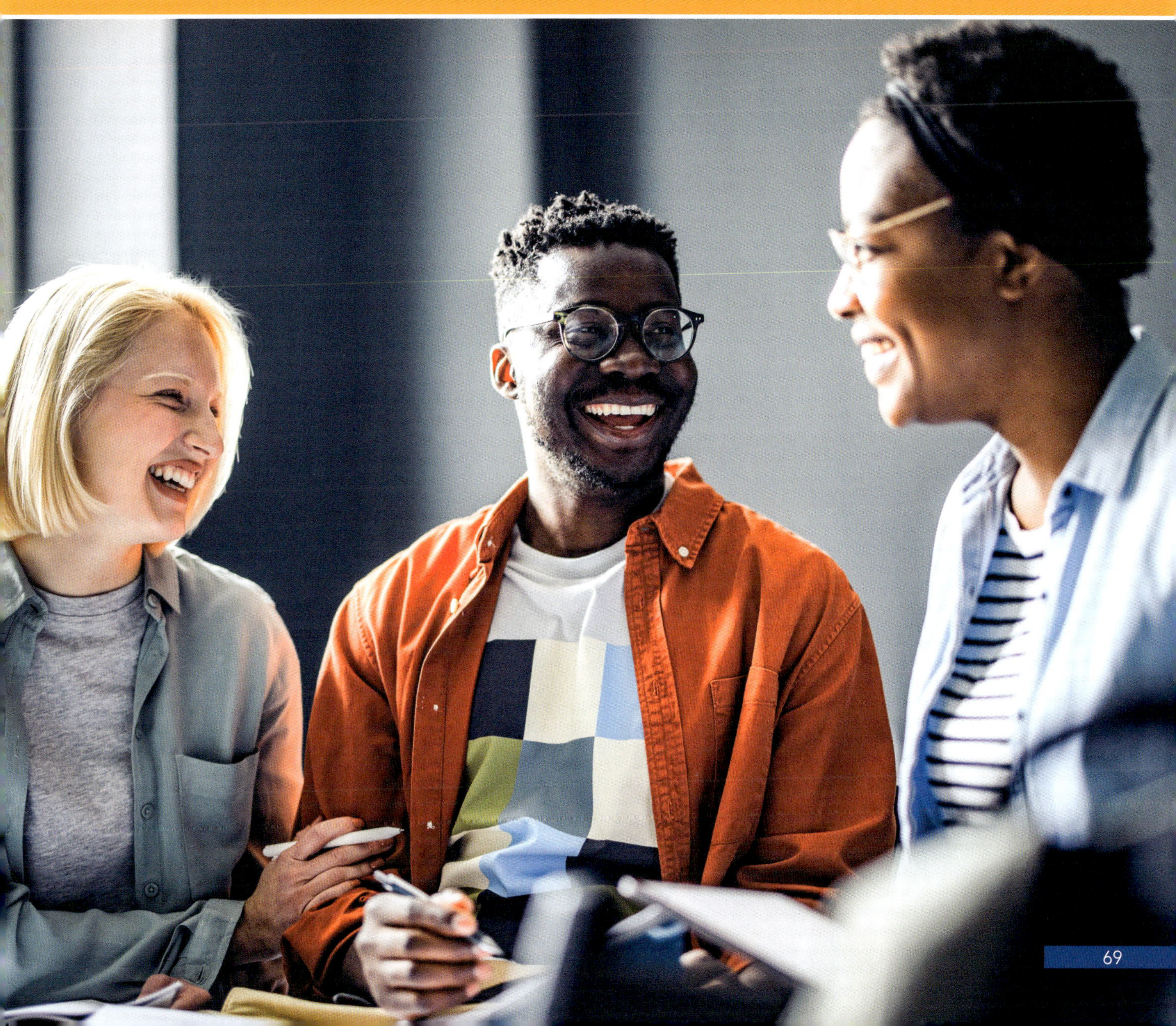

In 1995 the first edition of the National Health Education Standards was published by the Joint Committee for National Health Education Standards (see footnote) with support from the American Cancer Society, and over the following 10 years, 38 states adopted or adapted the National HE Standards for their use. The impact of the National HE Standards can be seen in policy and program changes at national, state, and local levels. In addition, all major health education curricula now reference these national standards. In 2003 the American Cancer Society (ACS) agreed to provide funding and staff support for the review, revision, and production of the standards (second edition).

"Never doubt that a small group of thoughtful, committed citizens can change the world. Indeed, it is the only thing that ever has."

Margaret Mead, quoted in Hellison (2011, p. 3)

Task Force

SHAPE America, the nation's largest organization serving and representing school-based health education professionals, obtained the copyright to the National HE Standards in 2020 when its longtime partner, the American Cancer Society, divested from the school health space. In spring 2021, through a call for task force members, leaders emerged who offered diverse perspectives and held deep content knowledge and experience in health education. They represented a variety of stakeholders in school-based health education, including leading national health education organizations, state departments of education, university health education teacher education (HETE) programs, and preK-12 practitioners.

Members and cochairs were selected during summer 2021, and in September the National HE Standards Task Force was formed and officially launched. The defined objective of this temporary group was to revise the second edition of the National HE Standards and develop a set of standards that advances the field of school-based health education.

Process to Revise the Standards

Six distinct steps provided an overarching road map for the National HE Standards Task Force efforts: Building Community, Vision, Standards Statements, Performance Indicators, Document, and Rollout and Implementation (see figures 7.1 and 7.2).

During the two-plus-year process, *Building Community* was foundational to the efforts of the National HE Standards Task Force. This early phase concentrated on establishing expectations, defining collaborative norms, consensus building, practicing conflict resolution, and identifying expertise. Next, the National HE Standards Task Force explored a shared *Vision* through performing a SWOT (strengths, weaknesses, opportunities, and threats) analysis of the second edition, creating a vision of attributes of a healthy person, identifying overarching themes, and investigating a variety of state and national standards in health and

The Joint Committee for National Health Education Standards was formed with members from the American Association for Health Education (AAHE—formerly the Association for the Advancement of Health Education), the American Public Health Association (APHA), the American School Health Association (ASHA), and the Society of State Directors of Health, Physical Education, and Recreation (SSDHPER).

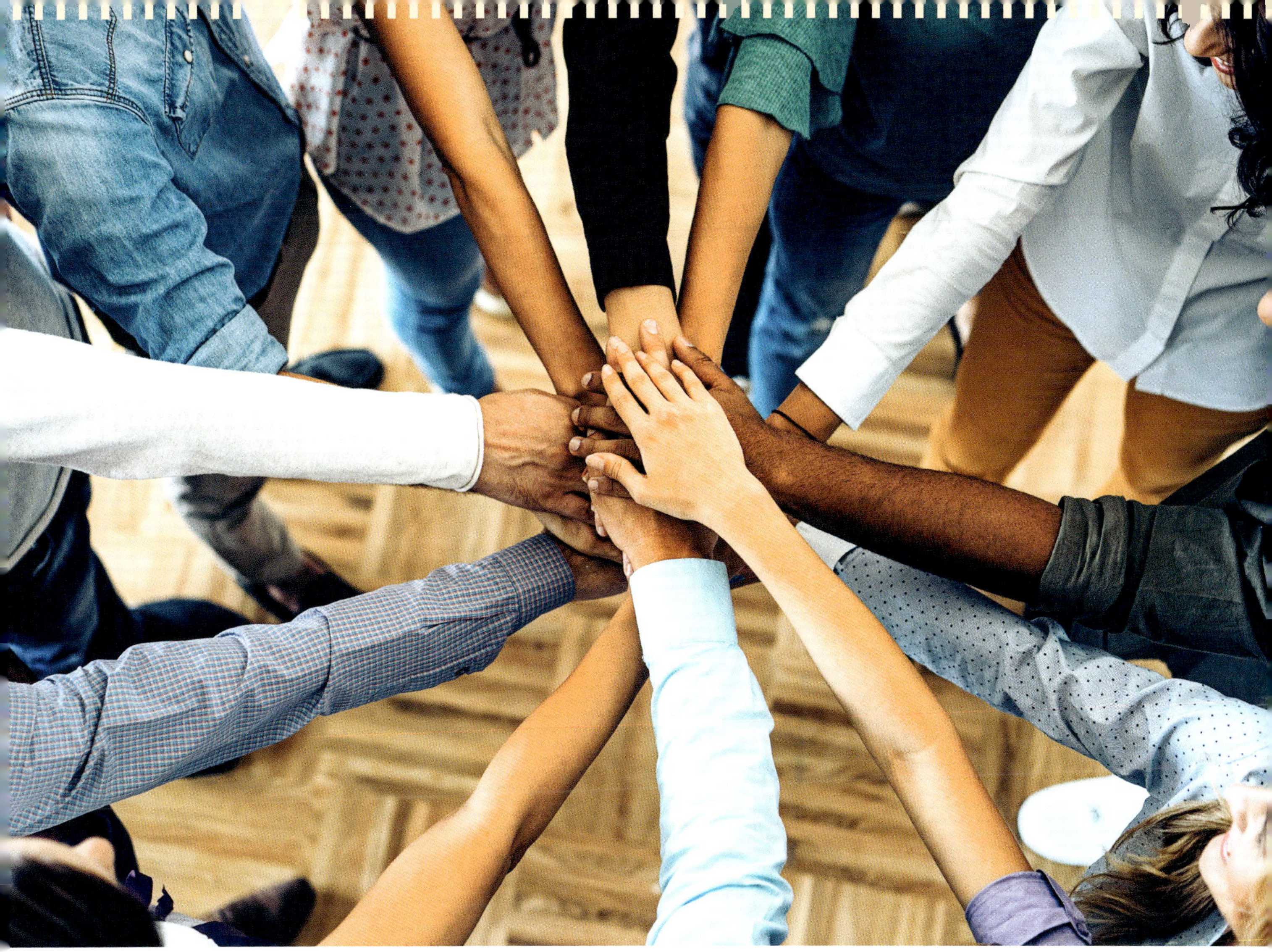

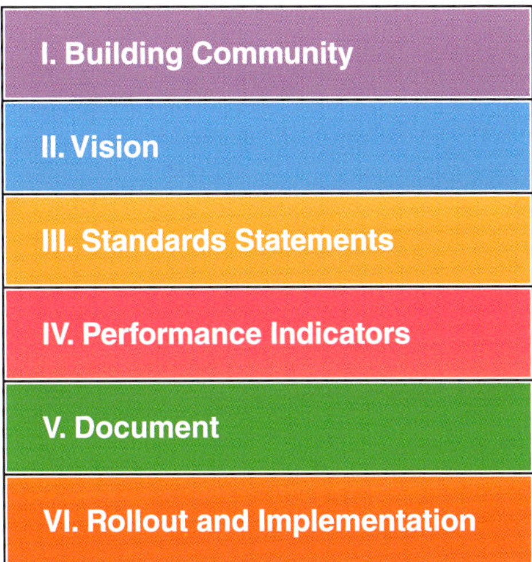

FIGURE 7.1 Task force road map for revision process.

National HE Standards Revision Timeline

2021

March through August	Called for nominations for National HE Standards Revision Task Force Selected Task Force members and cochairs Charged Task Force with revision of National HE Standards (second edition)
September through December	Task Force began regular meetings *Building Community:* Established collaborative norms, practiced consensus building and conflict resolution, identified expertise areas *Vision:* Discussed attributes of a healthy person, health education theory

2022

January through May	Investigated state and national standards in health and other content areas Reviewed town hall and survey feedback Attended SHAPE America National Convention: breakout sessions, coffee talks, survey Attended in-person work session in New Orleans, Louisiana
May through December	Debriefed convention feedback *Standards Statements:* Revised initial draft Participated in virtual summer retreat *Performance Indicators:* Reviewed horizontal and vertical alignments Revised initial draft of Standards, Rationales, and Performance Indicators

2023

January through May	Finalized initial draft of National HE Standards (third edition) Attended SHAPE America National Convention: breakout sessions, coffee talks Launched survey as first public review for National HE Standards (third edition) draft Hosted National HE Standards town hall to gather feedback
June through August	Revised initial draft of Standards, Rationales, and Performance Indicators based on stakeholder feedback and first public review Participated in virtual summer retreat Finalized National HE Standards (third edition) draft for second public review

September through December	Launched survey as second public review for National HE Standards (third edition) draft Revised and finalized National HE Standards (third edition) draft based on public review feedback *Document:* Finalized National HE Standards (third edition) for production and rollout

2024

January through March	Produced National HE Standards (third edition) *Rollout and Implementation:* Launched National HE Standards (third edition)

FIGURE 7.2 Task force timeline for revision process.

other content areas. Soon afterward, careful examination began of the *Standard Statements* and *Performance Indicators*. This review of each standard statement, rationale, and all related performance indicators was applied horizontally according to grade span for appropriateness and progression and also vertically for consistency and relevancy. Document revision incorporated edits informed by current theory, member expertise, and, most significantly, internal and external stakeholder feedback. Throughout the process, ongoing communication and stakeholder input was vital. A variety of methods for collecting both formal and informal feedback included virtual town hall meetings, podcasts, conference sessions, face-to-face coffee talks, and two rounds of public comment.

Using the feedback collected, revisions were made to the draft standards, rationale, and performance indicators. Along with their final versions, the *Document* manuscript was written to provide additional support and guidance for those using the standards in their practice.

APPENDIX A

Action Steps

Using the 2024 SHAPE America National Health Education Standards to make cross-curricular and interdisciplinary connections throughout the school environment allows for a coordinated approach to support school-based health education in meaningful ways among health education stakeholders. This appendix is divided into action steps for state education agencies, local education agencies, higher education, and national organizations and agencies to provide concrete actions that health education stakeholders can take to support the National Health Education Standards. For more details on how health educators can support meaningful standards-based health education, see chapter 4.

Implementation Action Steps for Higher Education

Coordinating Policy, Process, and Practice

- Explain how school policy is developed and the ramifications that occur in the classroom as a result (e.g., opting out of sexuality education lessons).
- Encourage students to volunteer to serve on policy committees and have a voice in the development of policy, process, and practice.
- Prepare students to be able to communicate the importance of cross-disciplinary articulation of health information and services through training, publications, and resources in physical education class, physical activity opportunities, and the nutrition environment and services.
- Model the use of technology as a tool for curriculum, instruction, and assessment in professional coursework to support the effective and critical use of technology by future and current teachers.
- Prepare preservice and in-service teachers to be student health education advocates, observing student progress and requesting all necessary instructional time and resources for learning mastery.
- Prepare students to be able to support cross-disciplinary articulation of health information and services through training, publications, and resources with school-based health services, including counseling and mental health services.

Professional Development

- Encourage higher education administrators to provide support and incentives to health education faculty who lead in-service training in standards implementation and assessment through school, university, and community partnerships.

- Promote teaching and research opportunities related to the National HE Standards and their assessment.
- Assist in preservice and in-service workshops for teachers who need support and experience with the synergistic effects of curriculum, instruction, and assessment.
- Expand the professional development of school health education faculty who promote the National HE Standards in their teaching, research, and service commitments

Curriculum and Instruction

- Show the relationship between teaching a skill in physical education and teaching a skill in health education.
- Provide adequate health education training for dual-licensure students.
- Model how to teach skills-based health in a physical education class.
- Prepare students to teach skills-based nutrition education.
- Develop courses that enhance preservice teachers' health education skills and competencies through the National HE Standards.
- Prepare future teachers to use a variety of instructional methods, strategies, technologies, and resources in health instruction to meet the learning styles, interests, and needs of a diverse student population.
- Prepare future teachers to integrate health-related concepts with skills across the preK-12 curriculum, as guided by the National HE Standards.
- Advocate for National HE Standards alignment in preK-12 curriculum development and deliberation at local, state, and national levels.
- Promote the design, use, and dissemination of standards-based, research-based curricula and programs in professional preparation coursework, internships, and fieldwork.
- Influence faculty in health education, teacher education, educational leadership, and educational psychology programs to prepare future school professionals to use the National HE Standards and to promote health as an essential element in academic achievement across the school curriculum.

Assessment

- Prepare future teachers to create or select and use a variety of authentic assessments (e.g., portfolio and performance) to achieve the National HE Standards.
- Assist in preservice and in-service workshops for teachers who need practice in assessing student work products in the context of their teaching practices and pedagogy.
- Provide leadership in linking research to practice in school health education.

Family and Community Involvement

- Train students to practice a variety of strategies to communicate with parents and caregivers.

- Encourage students to engage with and involve students in planning parent and caregiver education programs (e.g., newsletters).
- Prepare students to examine the community of their school and determine ways the community can support the skills-based health program.

Implementation Action Steps for Local Education Agencies (LEA)

Coordinating Policy, Process, and Practice

- Establish policies and provide supervision and support to ensure that health education is being implemented on the local level (ODPHP, n.d.).
- Require preK-12 health education to be taught by licensed health educators.
- Schedule instructional time sufficient to acquire health education content and skills, to actively participate in the learning, for students to practice skills, and to reflect.
- Provide teachers with the resources, dedicated learning space, and access to technology and equipment that they need to meet the goals of the National HE Standards.
- Designate a health education coordinator position to provide support to health educators through guidance, professional development, and technical assistance.
- Promote collaboration between the school nurse, counselors, mental health providers, and the health educator.

Professional Development

- Provide high-quality ongoing professional development in health education content, skills, and pedagogical practices.
- Provide adequate training for technology and use of equipment and resources.
- Provide ongoing professional development in student assessment and curriculum evaluation to health education teachers.
- Support teachers in planning, implementing, and aligning health instruction with the National HE Standards and/or state standards.

Curriculum and Instruction

- Implement a district-wide preK-12 comprehensive school health curriculum that is aligned with the National HE Standards and/or state standards.
- Create a scope and sequence that is based on the National HE Standards and that increases knowledge and skill development.
- Require that health education for preK-12 is responsive to developmental levels and a variety of learning styles.
- Administer the health education curriculum in a manner that is consistent with best practice recommendations from state and federal agencies and

professional education and health organizations (e.g., research based, unbiased, gender sensitive, multicultural, and focused on health needs and outcomes).

- Update and revise the district-wide health education curriculum, in alignment with the National HE Standards, on a regular revision cycle, with leadership from school principals and curriculum coordinators in collaboration with licensed or certified health educators.
- Identify opportunities for integration of National HE Standards performance indicators into physical education curriculum.
- Support cross-disciplinary articulation of health information and services through training, publications, and resources in physical education class, physical activity opportunities, and the nutrition environment and services.

Assessment

- Use authentic student assessments to determine whether the goals of the National HE Standards and/or state standards are being met.
- Require the reporting of student progress in health education.
- Provide ongoing professional development in student assessment and curriculum evaluation to health education teachers.

Family and Community Involvement

- Encourage ongoing parent or caregiver and community involvement in school health education programs.
- Encourage communication between the health education program and parents or caregivers and the community.

Implementation Action Steps for National Organizations and Agencies

Coordinating Policy, Process, and Practice

- Support state and local school systems in implementing standards-based health education in schools.
- Advocate with policymakers at local, state, and national levels to ensure all students have educational opportunities for preK-12 health education.
- Support coalitions of education, school health, and public health advocates and decision makers in order to elevate the need for increased support for school-based health education.
- Include health education pedagogical knowledge and skills in national teacher examination prior to licensure.
- Assist in the development of quality measures and accreditation standards for health education programs.

Professional Development

- Provide high-quality professional development programs for teachers, faculty, and other health professionals addressing effective student learning and skill acquisition.
- Support efforts to provide professional development for teachers, faculty, administrators, and other health professionals on quality health education.
- Support and advocate for licensed or certified health teachers to teach preK-12 health education.

Curriculum and Instruction

- Support and advocate for quality preK-12 health instruction in public, private, charter, and parochial schools.
- Support current research and provide support materials focused on quality health education for dissemination.
- Partner with other education and health organizations to support policies related to preK-12 comprehensive school health education and standards-based curricula, instruction, and assessment.

Family and Community Involvement

- Participate in coalitions of education, school health, and public health advocates, such as the local wellness committee, in order to highlight the need for increased support for school-based health education.

Implementation Action Steps for State Education Agencies (SEA)

Coordinating Policy, Process, and Practice

- Support the adoption of policies or regulations that ensure adequate instructional time for health education instruction (ODPHP, n.d.).
- Designate a health education leadership position within the SEA to provide statewide support to health educators through guidance, professional development, and technical assistance.
- Use student behavioral data, and the impact of those behaviors on learning, to support programs that enable students to reduce barriers to learning.
- Establish policies or regulations that identify health education as a required program of study, and establish a climate for successful program implementation.
- Provide support and technical assistance to LEA in the area of data collection and analysis relative to health education curricular decisions.
- Employ appropriately licensed or certified school health educators and specialists within SEA to provide leadership and assistance to local schools and communities.

- Support cross-disciplinary articulation of health information and services through training, publications, and resources with school-based health services, including counseling and mental health services.
- Set professional standards for teacher licensure in health education in collaboration with accreditation agencies and institutions.
- Require that highly qualified teacher standards, stated in federal legislation, be applied to health educators.
- Support cross-disciplinary articulation of health information and services through training, publications, and resources in physical education class, physical activity opportunities, and the nutrition environment and services.

Professional Development

- Ensure that high-quality professional learning, which includes work/study, collaboration, and professional development, occurs and is available for all teachers, curriculum specialists, and district leaders.
- Ensure that high-quality professional learning is aligned with the SEA's professional standards for teaching practices and with professional learning as defined by the National Staff Development Council.
- Provide teacher training and professional development with a focus on standards-based instruction, including guidance to schools on periodic monitoring of compliance and quality control issues.
- Promote differentiated instruction in professional development opportunities to meet the emotional, intellectual, physical, and social needs of all students.

Curriculum and Instruction

- Support LEA by promoting preK-12 health education curricula and programs that are consistent with best practice recommendations of state and federal agencies and professional education and health organizations.
- Provide LEA with curricular and instructional support materials, such as state standards, scope and sequence, alignment and mapping tools, and frameworks, that are needed to meet the National HE Standards and/or state standards.
- Where appropriate, guide LEA to adopt research-based health education curricula and programs that are aligned with the National HE Standards.

Assessment

- Provide LEA with ongoing assessment training in standards-based curricula so they can work with teachers and administrators to develop their own local assessments of students.
- Provide support to districts in writing, developing, and scoring authentic student assessments to determine whether the goals of the National HE Standards are being met.
- Develop and implement a statewide assessment program that addresses health knowledge and skills across the preK-12 curriculum.

Technology

- Provide electronic resources with standards-based sample instructional and assessment activities to teachers across the state.
- Implement and maintain a website for health education that provides links, updates, registrations, and resources in the state.
- Encourage and support schools through training and funding to use technology to extend and expand instructional capacity.
- Ensure that preK-12 health education is part of the state and local technology plans.
- Provide technology training and support for the delivery of standards-based curriculum, instruction, and assessment.
- Encourage local districts to adopt instructional materials that use diverse technology tools.

Family and Community Involvement

- Highlight communities that support comprehensive health education in schools.
- Provide grant resources that are designed to build community support, activities, and resources for healthy children and their families.

APPENDIX B

Healthy People 2030 Goals

The Healthy People 2030 goals outlined below highlight the significant role that school-based health education has in promoting health and well-being for children and adolescents (ODPHP, n.d.). As stated in chapter 1, health educators and health education stakeholders play a vital role in supporting the national goals of improving health and well-being, and the National HE Standards provide the framework for that critical instruction.

Health Education

- Increase the proportion of schools requiring students to take at least 2 health education courses from grade 6 to 12 (AH-R06)
- Increase the proportion of adolescents who get formal sex education before age 18 years (FP-08)

Healthful and Risk-Reduction Behaviors Promoted in School Health Education

PERSONAL HEALTH AND WELLNESS

- Increase the proportion of children who get sufficient sleep (EMC-03)
- Reduce the proportion of students in grades 9 through 12 who report sunburn (C-10)
- Increase the proportion of children and adolescents who communicate positively with their parents (EMC-01)
- Increase the proportion of adolescents who have an adult they can talk to about serious problems (AH-03)

FOOD AND NUTRITION

- Reduce the proportion of children and adolescents with obesity (NWS-04)

PHYSICAL ACTIVITY

- Reduce the proportion of children and adolescents with obesity (NWS-04)
- Increase the proportion of adolescents who walk or bike to get places (PA-11)
- Increase the proportion of adolescents who do enough muscle-strengthening activity (PA-07)
- Increase the proportion of adolescents who do enough aerobic physical activity (PA-06)
- Increase the proportion of adolescents who do enough aerobic and muscle-strengthening activity (PA-08)

SEXUAL HEALTH

- Increase the proportion of adolescents who think substance abuse is risky (SU-R01)
- Increase the proportion of adolescents who have never had sex (FP-04)
- Reduce pregnancies in adolescents (FP-03)
- Increase the proportion of adolescents who use birth control the first time they have sex (FP-07)
- Increase the proportion of adolescent females who used effective birth control the last time they had sex (FP-05)
- Increase the proportion of adolescent males who used a condom the last time they had sex (FP-06)
- Increase the proportion of adolescent females at risk for unintended pregnancy who use effective birth control (FP-11)

SAFETY

- Reduce gun carrying among adolescents (IVP-12)
- Reduce suicide attempts by adolescents (MHMD-02)
- Reduce suicidal thoughts in lesbian, gay, or bisexual high school students (LGBT-06)
- Reduce suicidal thoughts in transgender students (LGBT-D02)

MENTAL AND EMOTIONAL HEALTH

- Increase the proportion of children and adolescents who show resilience to challenges and stress (EMC-D07)
- Reduce suicidal thoughts in lesbian, gay, or bisexual high school students (LGBT-06)
- Reduce suicidal thoughts in transgender students (LGBT-D02)

ALCOHOL AND OTHER DRUGS

- Reduce the proportion of adolescents who drank alcohol in the past month (SU-04)
- Reduce the proportion of people under 21 years who engaged in binge drinking in the past month (SU-09)
- Reduce the proportion of adolescents who used drugs in the past month (SU-05)
- Reduce the proportion of adolescents who used marijuana in the past month (SU-06)
- Reduce the proportion of lesbian, gay, or bisexual high school students who have used illicit drugs (LGBT-07)
- Reduce the proportion of transgender high school students who have used illicit drugs (LGBT-D03)

TOBACCO

- Eliminate cigarette smoking initiation in adolescents and young adults (TU-10)

- Reduce the proportion of people who don't smoke but are exposed to secondhand smoke (TU-19)
- Reduce current tobacco use in adolescents (TU-04)
- Reduce current e-cigarette use in adolescents (TU-05)
- Reduce current cigarette smoking in adolescents (TU-06)
- Reduce current use of smokeless tobacco products among adolescents (TU-08)
- Reduce current use of flavored tobacco products in adolescents who use tobacco (TU-09)

VIOLENCE

- Reduce gun carrying among adolescents (IVP-12)
- Reduce physical fighting among adolescents (IVP-11)
- Reduce adolescent sexual violence by anyone (IVP-17)
- Reduce sexual or physical adolescent dating violence (IVP-18)
- Reduce bullying of lesbian, gay, or bisexual high school students (LGBT-05)
- Reduce bullying of transgender students (LGBT-D01)

Physical Education and Physical Activity

- Increase the proportion of child care centers where children aged 3 to 5 years do at least 60 minutes of physical activity a day (PA-R01)
- Increase the proportion of adolescents who participate in daily school physical education (ECBP-01)

Nutrition Environment and Services

- Increase the proportion of students participating in the School Breakfast Program (AH-04)
- Increase the proportion of schools that don't sell less healthy foods and drinks (ECBP-D02)
- Increase the proportion of eligible students participating in the Summer Food Service Program (AH-R03)

Health Services

- Increase the proportion of children aged 3 to 5 years who get vision screening (V-01)
- Increase use of the oral health care system (OH-08)
- Increase the proportion of middle and high schools that provide case management for chronic conditions (ECBP-D01)
- Increase the proportion of secondary schools with a full-time registered nurse (AH-R08)

Counseling, Psychological, and Social Services

- Increase the proportion of public schools with a counselor, social worker, and psychologist (AH-R09)

- Increase the proportion of children and adolescents with symptoms of trauma who get treatment (AH-D02)
- Increase the proportion of children and adolescents who get preventive mental health care in school (EMC-D06)
- Increase the proportion of children and adolescents with ADHD who get appropriate treatment (EMC-04)
- Increase the proportion of children with mental health problems who get treatment (MHMD-03)
- Increase the proportion of children and adolescents who get appropriate treatment for behavior problems (EMC-D05)
- Increase the proportion of children and adolescents who get appropriate treatment for anxiety or depression (EMC-D04)

Social and Emotional Climate

- Increase the proportion of trauma-informed early childcare settings and elementary and secondary schools (AH-D01)

Physical Environment

- Increase the proportion of schools with policies and practices that promote health and safety (EH-D01)
- Reduce the proportion of public schools with a serious violent incident (AH-D03)

Employee Wellness

- Reduce work-related assaults (OSH-05)
- Increase the proportion of worksites that offer an employee health promotion program (ECBP-D03)
- Increase the proportion of worksites that offer an employee physical activity program (ECBP-D04)
- Increase the proportion of worksites that offer an employee nutrition program (ECBP-D05)

Family Engagement

- Increase the proportion of children whose family read to them at least 4 days per week (EMC-02)
- Increase the proportion of parents and guardians who know the emergency or evacuation plan for their children's school (PREP-D01)
- Increase the proportion of parents who follow AAP recommendations on limiting screen time for children aged 6 to 17 years (PA-R02)

Community Involvement

- Reduce the proportion of adolescents and young adults who aren't in school or working (AH-09)
- Increase the proportion of schools with policies and practices that promote health and safety (EH-D01)

- Reduce the proportion of adolescents exposed to tobacco marketing (TU-22)
- Reduce the rate of adolescent and young adult victimization from violent crimes (AH-R1)
- Increase the proportion of children who receive a developmental screening (MICH-17)
- Increase the proportion of 4th-graders with math skills at or above the proficient level (AH-06)
- Increase the proportion of 4th-graders with reading skills at or above the proficient level (AH-05)
- Increase the proportion of 8th-graders with reading skills at or above the proficient level (AH-R04)
- Increase the proportion of 8th-graders with math skills at or above the proficient level (AH-R05)
- Increase the proportion of secondary schools with a start time of 8:30 AM or later (AH-R07)
- Reduce chronic school absence among early adolescents (AH-07)
- Reduce the proportion of adolescents and young adults who aren't in school or working (AH-09)
- Reduce the proportion of children and adolescents who are suspended or expelled (EMC-D02)
- Increase the proportion of high school students who graduate in 4 years (AH-08)

GLOSSARY

asset-based—Utilizing the strength and opportunities that the individual, family, or community provides rather than having a deficit focus.

assessment—The process of gathering, describing, or quantifying student learning as it relates to the established learning objective.

assessment cycle—The process of assessing student learning by establishing learning goals, designing assessment and instruction, gathering data on reaching the goal, and using the data to adjust or maintain instruction (Connolly, 2020).

authentic assessment—An evaluation of students that realistically measures the ability to apply knowledge and skills in real-world situations, settings, and contexts.

backward design—Process of planning that includes "data analysis, establishment of content and skill performance indicators, designing of assessment, then instruction" (Connolly, 2020, p. 48).

comprehensive school health education—Comprehensive school health education incorporates a structured, developmentally appropriate series of intended learning outcomes and associated learning experiences for students, including teaching strategies and learning experiences that provide students with opportunities to acquire the attitudes, knowledge, and skills necessary for making health-promoting decisions, generally organized as a detailed set of directions, strategies, lessons, and assessment (adapted from CDC, 2021).

culturally responsive—Culturally responsive means to use "the cultural knowledge, prior experiences, frames of reference, and performance styles of ethnically diverse students to make learning encounters more relevant to and effective for them" (Gay, 2018, p. 36).

curriculum—Curriculum is a set of plans for guiding student learning that serves as the basis for instruction in the classroom. Curriculum includes specific learning goals, content, strategies, assessment, and resources.

curriculum map—A visual representation of the skills, content, and assessments that are taught in a class, grade level, or program. It helps align the curriculum with 2024 National Health Education Standards, plan for instruction, and reflect on previous teaching and learning experiences.

curriculum planning—The process of making decisions about what to learn and why, and how to organize the teaching and learning process, taking into account existing requirements, standards, and available resources (UNESCO, n.d.).

developmentally appropriate—"Curriculum materials that are consistent with an individual's cognitive, mental, emotional, physical, moral, and social development" (CDC, 2021).

differentiated instruction—Implementing strategies and techniques to meet the needs of all learners in the classroom, including but not limited to modifications to content, instruction, assessment, and the learning environment.

dimensions of wellness—A variety of interdependent health-related categories that affect overall health and well-being. Dimensions may include cultural, emotional, environmental, financial, intellectual, occupational, physical, sexual, social, and spiritual.

disinformation—False information that is disseminated with the intent to mislead or deceive.

diversity—The differences among individuals and groups of people based on factors such as race, ethnicity, sex, gender identity and expression, age, socioeconomic status, class, language, culture, religion, sexual orientation, ability, and geographical area (CDC, 2021).

equity—*See* health equity.

feedback—Communication with students based on their attempts to reach the learning goal. Effective criterion-referenced feedback results in increased learning due to a better understanding of expectations (Connolly, 2020).

formative assessment—Ongoing assessment that measures student progress toward achieving performance indicators or learning outcomes.

functional health information—Concepts and information that are accurate, reliable, and relevant and relate directly to health-promoting skills and behaviors. Examples of functional information include accurate information about risks of health-related behaviors, internal and external influences on health-risk behaviors, and socially normative behaviors.

health—"Health is a state of complete physical, mental and social well-being and not merely the absence of disease or infirmity" (WHO, n.d.).

health disparities—"Differences in health outcomes and their causes among segments of the population as defined by social, demographic, economic, environmental, or geographic category" (CDC, 2021).

health equity—The freedom from bias in which everyone has a fair and just opportunity to attain their highest level of health. Health resources are distributed based on the specific needs of an individual or population (CDC, 2022).

health helper—An individual or resource that can support the ability to be healthy and well.

health literacy (individual and organizational)—"Health literacy is the ability to access, understand, appraise, apply and advocate for health information and services in order to maintain or enhance one's own lifelong health and the health of others" (SHAPE America, 2015).

health promotion—"Any planned combination of educational, political, environmental, regulatory, and organizational mechanisms that support actions and conditions of living conducive to the health of individuals, families, groups, and communities" (CDC, 2021).

health-related skills—"Abilities to translate knowledge and readiness into the performance of actions that enable students to deal with social pressures, avoid or reduce risk-taking behaviors, enhance and maintain personal health, and promote the health of others" (CDC, 2021).

inclusion—Act or practice of behaviors and social norms that ensure people feel welcome and are treated fairly.

instructional practices and strategies—Techniques used by teachers to engage learners in activities designed to develop knowledge and build skills to achieve learning objectives.

learning styles—Ways that learners think, relate to, interpret, or process new information and learning.

misinformation—False or inaccurate information conveyed without the intention of deliberately deceiving.

participatory teaching activities—A method that uses modeling, observation, and social interaction.

perceived susceptibility and perceived severity—Grounded in the health belief model, it is the likelihood of illness and injury (susceptibility) and a belief about the potential consequences (severity).

performance-based assessment—Evaluation that provides an opportunity for students to demonstrate their learning in authentic ways (SHAPE America, 2015). *See* authentic assessment.

performance indicators—Performance indicators articulate what a student should achieve by the end of a grade span. Achievement of performance indicators supports the successful attainment of the standard, increasing the likelihood of students adopting and maintaining healthy behaviors and enhancing health and well-being.

performance task—An authentic assessment consisting of a real-world, age-appropriate prompt, a corresponding rubric, and support materials, which the student needs to demonstrate proficiency (summative assessment) in Standard 1 and its paired skill performance indicator(s). May include but is not limited to role-plays, brochures, public service announcements, comic strips, songs, plays, and presentations to parents, principal, and staff (Connolly, 2020).

prompt—Directions given for an assessment task that explain criteria for success.

protective factor—"Assets (internal to individuals) and resources (external to individuals) that counteract, reduce, or eliminate the adverse effects of risk factors" (CDC, 2021).

reliable—The degree to which results of a measurement or process can be trusted to be accurate.

reliability—*See* reliable.

rubric—A guide used to score student work based on the criteria stated in the performance task or prompt.

scaffolding learning—Guidance or assistance provided to students with the goal of supporting their capacity of performing an activity or task, understanding the content, and gaining independence in the learning process (SHAPE America, 2015).

scope and sequence—An overview of the plan for instruction and format for seeing the overall picture of a detailed curriculum. It provides a plan for what learning should occur over the period of time covered and shows the scope of the material to be learned and practiced in what sequence. It also indicates how unit topics, skills, content knowledge, and culminating tasks build over time (Massachusetts Department of Elementary and Secondary Education, 2019).

skills-based health education—A planned, sequential, comprehensive, and relevant set of learning experiences implemented through socioecological and sociocultural perspectives and participatory methods, in order to support the development of skills, attitudes, and functional knowledge needed to maintain, enhance, or promote health and well-being of self and others across multiple dimensions of well-being (Benes & Alperin, 2022).

social determinants of health (SDOH)—Reflects "the conditions in the environments where people are born, live, learn, work, play, worship, and age that affect a wide range of health, functioning, and quality-of-life outcomes and risks." SDOH can be grouped into five domains: economic stability, education access and quality, health care access and quality, neighborhood and built environment, and social and community context (ODPHP, 2018).

social-emotional learning (SEL)—The "process through which all young people and adults acquire and apply the knowledge, skills, and attitudes to develop healthy identities, manage emotions and achieve personal and collective goals, feel and show empathy for others, establish and maintain supportive relationships, and make responsible and caring decisions" (CASEL, n.d.).

strength-based—*See* asset-based.

skills-based instruction—"A form of teaching that fosters classroom environments where critical thinking, collaboration, and active learning are developed at the same time as knowledge is acquired. A large portion of time is dedicated to practicing, assessing, and reflecting on skill development, and this instruction moves students toward independence and learning how to think critically and solve problems" (CDC, 2021).

student engagement—Degree to which students are interested in, paying attention to, curious about, invested in, and motivated by what and how they are learning (SHAPE America, 2015).

summative assessment—An assessment of learning, usually given at the end of an instructional unit, that measures achievement of the content and skill performance indicators such as role-play, projects, performance, and so on (Connolly, 2020).

universal design for learning (UDL)—Universal design for learning is a framework to improve and optimize teaching and learning for all people based on scientific insights into how humans learn. The three guidelines are the following: provide multiple means of engagement, provide multiple means of representation, and provide multiple means of action and expression (CAST, 2018).

valid—The quality of results to be credible, logical, and factual.

validity—*See* valid.

values—Principles, standards, and characteristics that represent what is most important to a person (Benes & Alperin, 2022).

well-being—Well-being is the combination of feeling good and functioning well; it is the experience of positive emotions such as happiness and contentment as well as the development of one's potential, having some control over one's life, having a sense of purpose, and experiencing positive relationships.

wellness—"A healthy state of balance among multiple dimensions of wellness, including the physical, social, emotional, mental, intellectual, spiritual, environmental, and occupational" (SHAPE America, 2015).

Whole School, Whole Community, Whole Child model (WSCC)—The WSCC model combines and builds on elements of the traditional coordinated school health approach and the whole child framework. It addresses the need for greater alignment, integration, and collaboration between education and health to improve each child's cognitive, physical, social, and emotional development by providing a framework to address the symbiotic relationship between learning and health (ASCD, 2024).

REFERENCES

American Cancer Society (2007). *National health education standards: Achieving excellence* (2nd ed.). American Cancer Society.

Antonovsky, A. (1996). The salutogenic model as a theory to guide health promotion. *Health Promotion International*, *11*(1), 11-18. https://doi.org/10.1093/heapro/11.1.11

ASCD. (2024). *The ASCD whole child approach to education*. www.ascd.org/whole-child

Association for Schools and Programs of Public Health on Racism and Public Health (ASPPH). (2020). *ASPPH statement: Racism is a public health crisis*. https://s3.us-east-1.amazonaws.com/ASPPH_Media_Files/Docs/Final%20ASPPH%20Statement%20on%20racism.pdf

Beale-Tawfeeq, A.K., Anderson, A., and Ramos, W.D. (2018). A cause to action: Learning to develop a culturally responsive/relevant approach to 21st century water safety messaging through collaborative partnerships. *International Journal of Aquatic Research and Education*, *11*(1), Article 8. https://doi.org/10.25035/ijare.11.01.08

Beale-Tawfeeq, A.K., Waller, S.N., and Quash, T.M. (2023). Third diversity in aquatics special issue. *International Journal of Aquatic Research and Education*, *14*(2), Article 3. https://doi.org/10.25035/ijare.14.02.03

Berg, C.J., Callaghan, W.M., Syverson, C., & Henderson, Z. (2010, December). Pregnancy-related mortality in the United States, 1998 to 2005. *Obstetrics & Gynecology, 116*(6), 1302-1309. https://doi.org/10.1097/AOG.0b013e3181fdfb11

Benes, S. (2020). Health education as a social justice tool. In S. Brand & L. Ciccomascolo (Eds), *Social justice and putting theory into practice in schools and communities* (pp. 58-80). IGI Global.

Benes, S., & Alperin, H. (2022). *Essentials of teaching health education: Curriculum, instruction and assessment* (2nd ed.). Human Kinetics.

Benes, S., & Alperin, H. (2023). Health education: Concepts, professions, and issues. In D. Siedentop & H. van der Mars (Eds.), *Introduction to physical education, fitness, and sport* (9th ed., pp. 415-449). Human Kinetics.

Bhattacharya, S., Pradhan, K.B., Bashar, M.A., Tripathi, S., Thiyagarajan, A., Srivastava, A., & Singh, A. (2020). Salutogenesis: A bona fide guide towards health preservation. *Journal of Family Medicine and Primary Care*, *9*(1), 16-19. https://doi.org/10.4103/jfmpc.jfmpc_260_19

Blackshear, T., & Culp, B. (2020): Transforming PETE's initial standards: Ensuring social justice for Black students in physical education. *Quest*, *73*(1), 22-44. https://doi.org/10.1080/00336297.2020.1838305

Boyer, E.L. (1990). *A special report. Scholarship reconsidered: Priorities of the professoriate*. The Carnegie Foundation for the Advancement of Teaching.

Bröder, J., Okan, O., Bauer, U., et al. (2017). Health literacy in childhood and youth: A systematic review of definitions and models. *BMC Public Health*, *17*, 361. https://doi.org/10.1186/s12889-017-4267-y

Brookhart, S.M. (2024). *Classroom assessment essentials*. ASCD.

Cabrera, J.C., Rodriguez, M.C., Karl, S.R., & Chavez, C. (2018, April). *In what ways do health behaviors impact academic performance: Educational aspirations and commitment to learning?* [Conference presentation]. Annual meeting of the American Educational Research Association, New York, NY.

Canadian Healthy Schools Alliance. (2021). *Canadian healthy school standards*. www.healthyschoolsalliance.ca/en/resources

Carr, J.F., & Harris, D.E. (2001). *Succeeding with standards: Linking curriculum, assessment, and action planning*. Association for Supervision and Curriculum Development.

Collaborative for Academic, Social, and Emotional Learning (CASEL). (n.d.). SEL: What are the core competence areas and where are they promoted? https://casel.org/sel-framework/

CAST. (2018). *Universal design for learning guidelines version 2.2*. www.cast.org/impact/universal-design-for-learning-udl

CCSSO-SCASS Health Education Assessment Project. (2006). *Assessment tools for school health education, pre-service and in-service edition*. ToucanEd.

Centers for Disease Control and Prevention (CDC). (2014). *CDC healthy schools: Whole School, Whole Community, Whole Child (WSCC)*. www.cdc.gov/healthyschools/wscc/index.htm

Centers for Disease Control and Prevention (CDC). (2019). *Characteristics of effective health education curriculum*. www.cdc.gov/healthyschools/sher/characteristics/

Centers for Disease Control and Prevention (CDC). (2021). *Health education curriculum analysis tool (HECAT)—appendix 7*. www.cdc.gov/healthyyouth/HECAT/index.htm

Centers for Disease Control and Prevention (CDC). (2023, September 18). *Racism and Health*. https://cdc.gov/minorityhealth/racism-disparities/index.html

Centers for Disease Control and Prevention (CDC). (2022, July 1). *What is health equity?* Centers for Disease Control and Prevention. https://cdc.gov/healthequity/whatis/index.html

Centers for Disease Control and Prevention (CDC). (2023, February 9). *Whole School, Whole Community, Whole Child (WSCC)*. www.cdc.gov/healthyschools/wscc/index.htm

Clemens, T., Moreland, B., & Lee, R. (2021). Persistent racial/ethnic disparities in fatal unintentional drowning rates among persons aged ≤29 years—United States, 1999–2019. *Morbidity and Mortality Weekly Report, 70*, 869–874. http://dx.doi.org/10.15585/mmwr.mm7024a1external

Cochran-Smith, M. (2004). *Walking the road: Race, diversity, and social justice in teacher education*. New York, NY: Teachers College Press.

Connolly, M. (2019). *Skills-based health education*. Jones & Bartlett Learning.

Connolly, M. (2020). *Skills-based health education* (2nd ed.). Jones & Bartlett Learning.

Cosentino, G. (2016). *Indigenous peoples have a right to quality education. But so far, we've failed them*. World Economic Forum. https://weforum.org/agenda/2016/08/indigenous-people-have-a-right-to-quality-education-but-so-far-we-ve-failed-them/

Culp, B. (2021). Everyone matters: Eliminating dehumanizing practices in physical education. *Journal of Physical Education, Recreation & Dance, 92*(1), 19-26. https://doi.org/10.1080/07303084.2020.1838362

Delpit, L. (2013). *Multiplication is for white people: Raising expectations for other people's children*. New Press.

Frey, D.F. (2022, April 1). *Getting GREAT at feedback*. www.ascd.org/el/articles/getting-great-at-feedback

Gay, G. (2018). *Culturally responsive teaching: Theory, research, and practice* (3rd ed.). Teachers College Press.

Hellison, D. (2011). *Teaching responsibility through physical activity*. Human Kinetics.

Hess, K. (2023). *Rigor by design, not chance: Deeper thinking through actionable instruction and assessment*. Association for Supervision and Curriculum Development.

Ickovics, J.R., Carroll-Scott, A., Peters, S.M., Schwartz, M., Gilstad-Hayden, K., & McCaslin, I. (2014). Health and academic achievement: Cumulative effects of health assets on standardized test scores among urban youth. *Journal of School Health, 84*(1), 40-48. https://doi.org/10.1111/josh.12117

Institute of Education Sciences. (2023). *Fact sheet: Making sense of educational assessment*. Regional Educational Laboratory Northeast & Islands.

Jacobs, H.H. (2004). Development of a prologue: Setting the stage for curriculum mapping. In *Getting Results with Curriculum Mapping* (pp. 1-9). Association for Supervision and Curriculum Development.

Joint Committee on National Health Education Standards. (2007). *National health education standards: Achieving excellence* (2nd ed.). American Cancer Society.

Kendi, S., & Macy, M.L. (2023). The injury equity framework—establishing a unified approach for addressing inequities. *The New England Journal of Medicine, 388*(9), 774-776. https://doi.org/10.1056/NEJMp2212378

Killen, M., & Rutland, A. (2022). Promoting fair and just school environments: Developing inclusive youth. *Policy Insights From the Behavioral and Brain Sciences, 9*(1), 81-89. https://doi.org/10.1177/23727322211073795

Krawec, P. (2022). *An indigenous call to unforgetting the past and reimagining our future*. Broadleaf Books.

Learning for Justice. (n.d.). Social just standards. www.tolerance.org/frameworks/social-justice-standards

Lewallen, T.C., Hunt, H., Potts-Datema, W., Zaza, S., & Giles, W. (2015, November). The whole school, whole community, whole child model: A new approach for improving educational attainment and healthy development for students. *Journal of School Health, 85*(11),729-739. https://doi: 10.1111/josh.12310; PMID: 26440815; PMCID: PMC4606766

Lovett-Scott, M., & Prather, F. (2014). *Global health systems: Comparing strategies for delivering health services*. Jones & Bartlett Learning.

Lumio. (2023, August). *Deliver engaging lessons—no matter where your learners are*. www.smarttech.com/en/lumio

Massachusetts Department of Elementary and Secondary Education. (2019). *Components of curriculum*. www.doe.mass.edu/acls/frameworks/components.html.

McTighe, J. (2005). Seven practices for effective learning. *Educational Leadership, 63*(3), 10-17.

McTighe, J., & Brown, P. (2020). Standards are not curriculum: Using understanding by design to make standards come alive. *Science and Children, 58*(1), 76-83.

Mentimeter. (2023, August). *Make your teaching count*. www.mentimeter.com

Michael, S.L., Merlo, C.L., Basch, C.E., Wentzel, K.R., & Wechsler, H. (2015). Critical connections: Health and academics. *Journal of School Health, 85*, 740-758.

Microsoft. (2023, August). *Flip*. https://info.flip.com/en-us.html

Mucedola, M. (2023). *Culture-based differentiated instruction: A guide to teaching health education* (1st ed.). Cognella Publishing

Mural. (2023, August). *Make it a Mural, not just a meeting*. www.mural.co

Myron Dueck, B.A. (2022, April 1). *Fine-tuning assessments for better feedback*. www.ascd.org/el/articles/fine-tuning-assessments-for-better-feedback

National Center on Deaf-Blindness. (n.d.). *Receptive and expressive communication*. www.nationaldb.org/media/doc/ReceptiveExpressiveCommunication_Wjlpsmp.pdf

Near Pod. (2023, July). *So many tools, so little time. Make any lesson interactive within one platform*. https://nearpod.com/streamline

Office of Disease Prevention and Health Promotion (ODPHP). (n.d.). *Healthy People 2030*. U.S. Department of Health and Human Services. https://health.gov/healthypeople/objectives-and-data/browse-objectives

Office of Disease Prevention and Health Promotion (ODPHP). (2018). *Healthy People 2030: Social determinants of health.* U.S. Department of Health and Human Services. https://health.gov/healthypeople/priority-areas/social-determinants-health

Office of Elementary and Secondary Education. (2016). *Non-regulatory guidance: Student support and academic achievement grants*. U.S. Department of Education. https://www2.ed.gov/policy/elsec/leg/essa/index.html

Penuel, W.R., Fishman, B.J., Cheng, B.H., & Sabelli, N. (2011). Organizing research and development at the intersection of learning, implementation, and design. *Educational Researcher*, 40, 331-337.

Persaud, A., Bhugra, D., Valsraj, K., & Bhavsar, V. (2021). Understanding geopolitical determinants of health. *Bulletin of the World Health Organization*, *99*(2), 166-168. https://doi.org/10.2471/BLT.20.254904

Popham, W.J. (2008). *Transformative assessment.* Association for Supervision and Curriculum Development.

Rasberry, C.N., Tiu, G.F., Kann, L., et al. (2015). Health-related behaviors and academic achievement among high school students—United States, 2015. Morbidity and Mortality Weekly Report, 66, 921-927.

Saphier, J., Haley-Speca, M.A., & Gower, R.R. (2017). *The skillful teacher: The comprehensive resource for improving teaching and learning* (7th ed.). Research for Better Teaching.

Sensoy, Ö., & Diangelo, R. (2009). Developing social justice literacy: An open letter to our faculty colleagues. *The Phi Delta Kappan*, *90*(5), 345-352. https://doi.org/10.1177/003172170909000508

SHAPE America – Society of Health and Physical Educators. (2015). *Appropriate practices in school-based health education*. [Guidance document]. SHAPE America.

SHAPE America – Society of Health and Physical Educators. (2018). *Health education is a critical component of a well-rounded education.* [Position Statement]. https://shapeamerica.org/Common/Uploaded%20files/document_manager/advocacy/position-statements/HE_Critical_Component_Position_Statement.pdf

SHAPE America – Society of Health and Physical Educators. (2025). *National Health Education Standards* (3rd ed.). SHAPE America.

SHAPE America – Society of Health and Physical Educators. (2022). *Social justice in PETE/HETE*. [Guidance document]. SHAPE America.

Tai, D.B.G., Sia, I.G., Doubeni, C.A., & Wieland, M.L. (2022). Disproportionate impact of COVID-19 on racial and ethnic minority groups in the United States: A 2021 update. *Journal of Racial and Ethnic Health Disparities*, *9*(6), 2334-2339. https://doi.org/10.1007/s40615-021-01170-w

Teisberg, E., Wallace, S., & O'Hara, S. (2020). Defining and implementing value-based health care: A strategic framework. *Academic Medicine: Journal of the Association of American Medical Colleges*, *95*(5), 682-685. https://doi.org/10.1097/ACM.0000000000003122

UNESCO. (n.d.). *Transforming curriculum today to build the education of tomorrow*. www.ibe.unesco.org/en

U.S. Department of Justice, Civil Rights Division. (2023). *Nondiscrimination on the basis of race, color, national origin, sex, religion, or age in law enforcement programs, services, and activities receiving assistance from the United States Department of Justice*. www.justice.gov/crt/nondiscrimination-basis-race-color-national-origin-sex-religion-or-age-law-enforcement-programs

U.S. Equal Employment Opportunity Commission. (2023). *Who is protected from employment discrimination?* www.eeoc.gov/employers/small-business/3-who-protected-employment-discrimination

Wiggins, G., & McTighe, J. (2005). *Understanding by design* (expanded 2nd ed.). Association for Supervision and Curriculum Development.

Wolfe, P. (2001). *Brain matters: Translating research into classroom practice*. ASCD.

World Health Organization (WHO). (n.d.). *Health and well-being*. www.who.int/data/gho/data/major-themes/health-and-well-being

World Health Organization (WHO). (2019). *Health promoting schools*. https://www.who.int/health-topics/health-promoting-schools

PHOTO CREDITS

Page 1: SDI Productions/E+/Getty Images
Page 3: SDI Productions/E+/Getty Images
Page 7: Hispanolistic/E+/Getty Images
Page 12: monkeybusinessimages/iStock/Getty Images Plus
Page 15: SDI Productions/E+/Getty Images
Page 17: FatCamera/E+/Getty Images
Page 18: FG Trade/E+/Getty Images
Page 20: Iparraguirre Recio/Moment/Getty Images
Page 23: Inside Creative House/iStock/Getty Images Plus
Page 37: Maskot/Maskot/Getty Images
Page 38: monkeybusinessimages/iStock/Getty Images Plus
Page 49: kali9/E+/Getty Images
Page 51: Drazen Zigic/iStock/Getty Images Plus
Page 69: miniseries/E+/Getty Images
Page 71: pixelfit/E+/Getty Images
Page 103: Courtesy of Kennesaw University; Courtesy of University of New Hampshire

ABOUT THE WRITERS

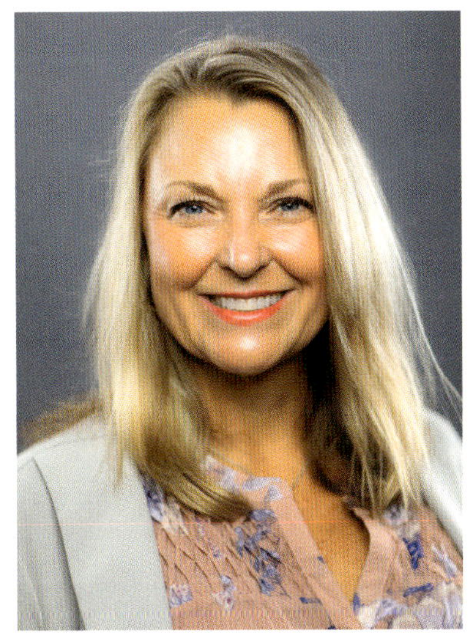

Kandice Porter, PhD, MCHES©, is a professor and associate dean for academic affairs in the Wellstar College of Health and Human Services at Kennesaw State University. She received both her bachelor's and master's degrees in health science education from the University of Florida and a doctorate in health behavior from Indiana University–Bloomington. Her teaching and research focus on effective pedagogical approaches in school health education. She works with national, state, and local organizations to promote quality school health efforts. In addition, she has been instrumental in developing degree programs in public health and integrated health sciences, as well as interprofessional coursework and research opportunities, within the Wellstar College.

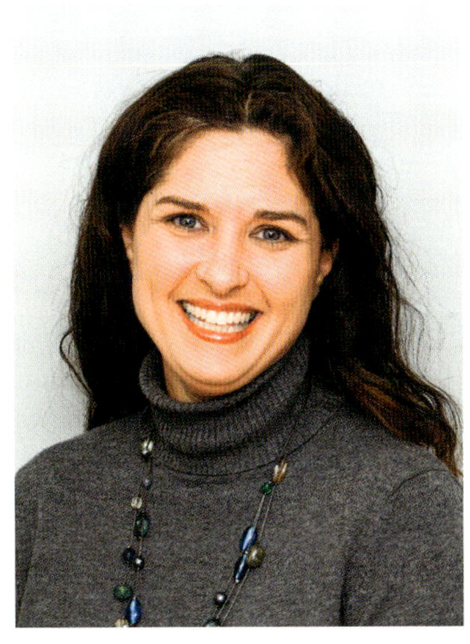

Holly Alperin, EdM, MCHES©, is a clinical associate professor at the University of New Hampshire (UNH) and has over 20 years of experience in both public health and education. As a faculty member and program coordinator of the department of kinesiology's health and physical education teacher preparation program, she focuses on preparing preservice educators to teach using a skills-based approach. Prior to UNH, she worked at the Massachusetts Department of Elementary and Secondary Education in a variety of roles that supported schools in their efforts to strengthen policies and increase capacity around school health education and programs, school nutrition programs, and professional learning experiences for educators. Alperin is the past vice president of health education for the New Hampshire Association for Health, Physical Education, Recreation and Dance as well as the past chair of SHAPE America's Health Education Council. She received her master's degree in education in policy, planning, and administration from Boston University and her bachelor's degree in health education and health promotion from Central Michigan University. She holds the Master Certified Health Education Specialist (MCHES) credential.

Angela Beale-Tawfeeq, PhD, MPH, has over 20 years of experience at the university level at various institutions, including Adelphi University, West Chester University, and Temple University. She is currently an associate professor of health and physical education teacher education at Rowan University. She has authored or coauthored many publications, including *Informal and Formal Mentoring for and by Scholars and Faculty of Color*, *Challenges and Strategies of Being an African American Chairperson in Kinesiology*, and *A Cause to Action: Learning to Develop a Culturally Responsive/Relevant Approach to 21st Century Water Safety Messaging Through Collaborative Partnerships*. Beale-Tawfeeq is the recipient of the 2021 SHAPE America E.B. Henderson Award. In her work, she strives to help individuals see the overall impact of social construct on the view of health and wellness.

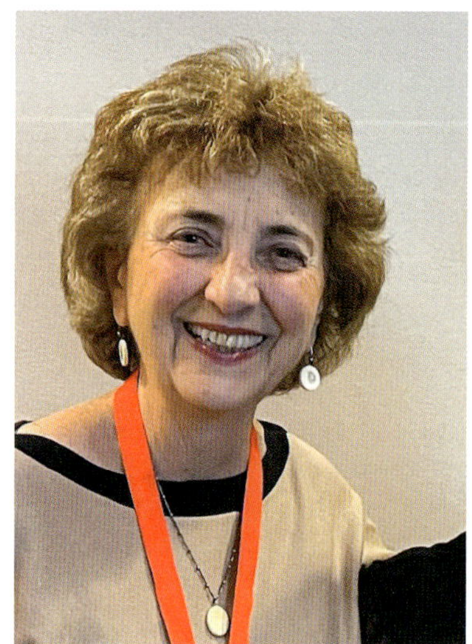

Mary Connolly, MEd, CHES©, is an adjunct professor at Curry College and a professor at Cambridge College. She is an accomplished health education professional whose career spans nearly four decades and includes teaching and administration in public schools and higher education. She served on the committee to revise the National Health Education Standards in 2007 and is a member of the Massachusetts Interdisciplinary Health Education and Human Services Advisory Council and the American School Health Association (ASHA) Coordinator's Committee. She is a reviewer for the National Council for Accreditation of Teacher Education. She was awarded the SHAPE America Lifetime Achievement Award in 2021.

ABOUT SHAPE AMERICA

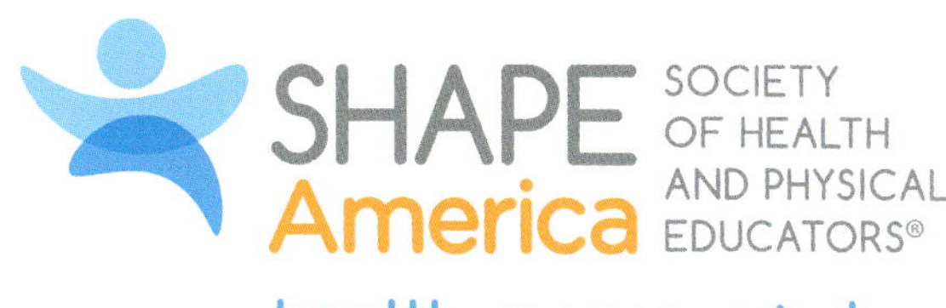

SHAPE America – Society of Health and Physical Educators serves as the voice for more than 200,000 health and physical education professionals across the United States. The organization's extensive community includes a diverse membership of health and physical educators, as well as advocates, supporters, and over 50 state affiliate organizations.

Since its founding in 1885, the organization has defined excellence in physical education. For decades, SHAPE America's National Standards for K-12 Physical Education have served as the foundation for well-designed physical education programs across the country, just as SHAPE America's National Health Education Standards serve as the foundation for effective skills-based health education. Together, these national standards provide a comprehensive framework for educators to deliver high-quality instruction and make a positive difference in the health and well-being of every preK-12 student.

SHAPE America provides programs, resources, and advocacy that support an inclusive, active, and healthier school culture, and the organization's newest program—health. moves. minds.©—helps teachers and schools incorporate social and emotional learning so students can thrive physically and emotionally.

Our Vision

A nation where all children are prepared to lead healthy, physically active lives.

Our Mission

To advance professional practice and promote research related to health and physical education, physical activity, dance, and sport.

To learn more, visit **www.shapeamerica.org**.

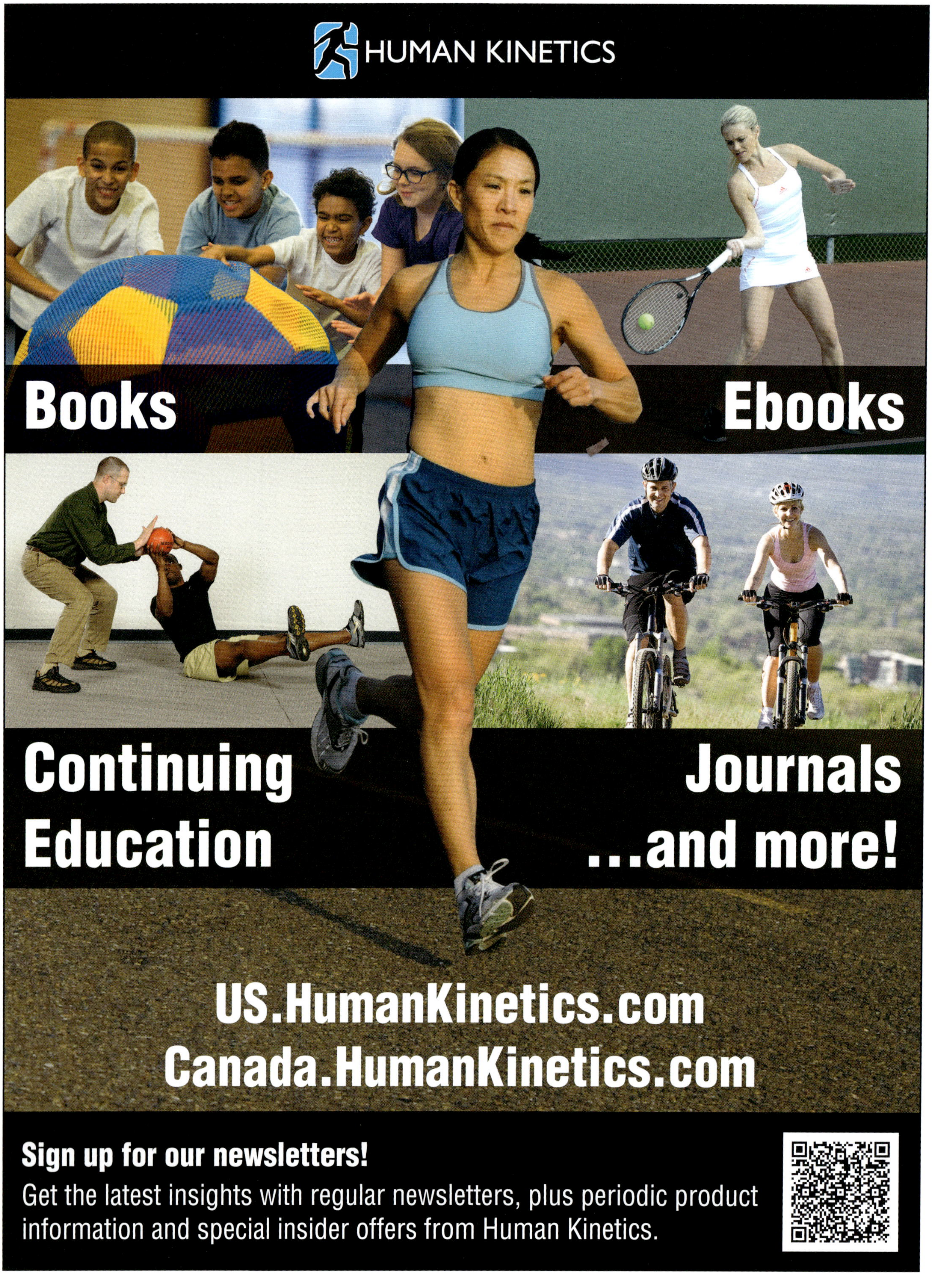

National Health Education Standards

THIRD EDITION

SHAPE AMERICA –
SOCIETY OF HEALTH AND PHYSICAL EDUCATORS